Smart Guide
to
Back Care

Smart Guide
to
BACK CARE

by Janet Wakley

Consultant Advisor
Dr Hans Mathew

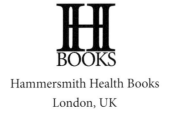

Hammersmith Health Books
London, UK

First published in 2012 by Hammersmith Health Books – an imprint of
Hammersmith Books Limited
14 Greville Street, London EC1N 8SB, UK
www.hammersmithbooks.co.uk

British Library Cataloguing in Publication Data: A CIP record of this book is
available from the British Library.

ISBN 978-1-78161-000-8
E-book ISBN: 978-1-78161-001-5
Commissioning editor: Georgina Bentliff
Designed and typeset by: Julie Bennett
Index: Dr Laurence Errington
Production: Helen Whitehorn, Pathmedia
Printed and bound by TJ International Ltd
Cover image: © Frederic Cirou/PhotoAlto/Corbis

Contents

Acknowledgements

I am indebted to Dr Hans Mathew for both his foreword and valuable support in the editing of this book. My thanks also to Mr Enrico Garofalo, photographer, and Mrs Laura Mullen, my model, for their time and assistance, as well as Miss Sarover Aujla, who helped with the early planning of the illustrations. I am also very grateful to Mr Robin Mugridge, whose extensive computer skills helped me with the compilation. Lastly, this book would not have been written if it were not for the patience and understanding of my husband, John, while I shut myself away for hours to do the writing.

About the Author

Janet Wakley's 28 years' experience as a registered nurse, specialising in post-anaesthetic recovery, included being an instructor and back care advisor to other medical staff. This focused on the safe moving and handling of patients and equipment within the hospital setting for the prevention of back injuries within the workplace. She now gives back care training to St John Ambulance Brigade members to help ensure their safe practice when out on duty. In addition, her own experience of back pain has ensured the methods and techniques that she promotes are those she uses herself within the context of her own busy lifestyle, in which nursing, bringing up a family and sport, including horse-riding, have all taken their toll.

Foreword

Having known Janet for the last 16 years and been first taught the basics of 'moving and handling' by her, I consider it an honour to write the foreword to her book. As a pain physician, I have treated many patients with back pain but unfortunately had the misfortune personally to shoulder a lifetime of low back pain from a childhood disability. I found reading this book useful, rewarding and gratifying, both in my personal life and professionally.

Global statistics on the incidence and causes of back pain vary greatly for multi-factorial reasons. In the UK, coming second only to the common cold, back pain is the highest reason for patients to seek medical advice, accounting for almost seven million GP visits annually. Experts estimate that as many as 80% of the population (that is four out of five people) will experience a back problem at some time in their lives. Most cases of back pain are mechanical or non-organic in origin. This means that they are not caused by serious conditions such as arthritis, infection, fracture or cancer.

The lower back is responsible for supporting most of the body's weight, therefore making it particularly vulnerable to strain and damage. The incidence of back problems is set to rise significantly in future years due to the population becoming increasingly obese.

Presented in a clear comprehensive style, the *Smart Guide to Back Care* is accessibly written, keeping medical jargon to a minimum. It presents a holistic approach to back problems, especially those arising in the home environment, where these are on the increase due to our sedentary lifestyles. This book empowers you to take control of your back; it places emphasis on using posture, positioning and exercises to ease, relieve and prevent back problems.

The initial chapters concentrate on the basic concepts of 'back care', progressing onto causes, risk assessment, moving and handling, prevention, better ways of daily movements, activities and strategic exercises for back strengthening and long-term pain relief and prevention of recurrence. The final few chapters describe treatment modalities including orthodox medical management and complementary therapies, all these again explained in simple terms.

There are many books on back pain available in the market, but this book is probably the only one that analyses the reasons for, and prevention and management of, back pain in the home surroundings. As a back pain sufferer I enjoyed and gained from reading this book and wish you also to have the same experience.

Dr Hans Mathew MBBS, MD, DA(UK), FFARCSI, MFPMRCA, DipMedAc

Chapter 1

Introduction

Global statistics on back pain vary greatly, but it is a fact that 19 out of 20 of us will get back pain at some time in our lives. The figures are staggering and the pain and discomfort experienced can be excruciating. Back pain in the UK is claimed to be the next most common ailment to the common cold and whereas we don't visit the doctor for colds, nearly seven million of us in the UK attend our surgeries, hobbling and grimacing with pain and spasm in our backs.

The NHS of England now estimates that the treatment of back pain costs around £481 million a year with nearly another £2 million spent on prescriptions and referrals for private consultations. In the USA, it is estimated to be in excess of $50 billion a year. But whatever the financial cost to the countries of the world, by any standard it is colossal, and the pain and prolonged discomfort of back pain are something we all wish to avoid.

In industry, British government legislation, under the Health and Safety at Work Act, 1974, requires employers to provide training in 'Moving and Handling' methods in order to protect their workers. This includes providing safe methods of work in a safe and healthy workplace. Under this legislation, the Manual Handling Operations Regulations 1992 further set out the responsibilities for both the employer and employee in respect of safe practice. This means that it is not just the responsibility of the employer to provide protection against injury, but also that the employee follows the guidelines provided within formal training sessions, to ensure that the work is carried out in a safe manner. If this were not enough, the Provision and Use of Work Equipment Regulations 1998 and the Lifting Operations and Lifting Equipment Regulations 1998 have also been produced in order to safeguard people from injury.

This is not just for manual workers either; the physical protection of all employees is now necessary. Consideration must now be given to things like the correct height of computer screens, well-designed chairs and work-stations, and the positioning of heavy boxes of stock or catering equipment.

The reason for all this government legislation in relation to the work environment is, of course, obvious. Back pain and muscle injury, as we all know, do not disappear overnight and many days off work reduce productivity and are an economic drain on the country. Statistics show that 50 million days of absence are as a result of work-related back injuries. That, in layman's terms, is roughly equivalent to 208,000 workers off sick for a whole year and costs businesses in England an estimated £5 billion. One can only imagine the statistics across the world. With approximately 40% of all adults experiencing an episode of back pain in a single year, about 40% of these will have symptoms that may last for several months. When an employee goes off sick with back pain, there is up to a 10% chance that they will still be off work a year later.

In the nursing profession alone (my profession), it is estimated that 80,000 British nurses a year suffer back injury during the course of their work and the numbers are not diminishing. This is despite the provision of a variety of equipment for use within the hospital setting and mandatory training sessions on moving and handling for all staff.

Back pain is not confined to employees or people over a certain age. Injury can occur to anyone and at any age. Yes, even teenagers. Back pain can affect every aspect of our daily activities and can bring with it a weakness that may render us more likely in the future to repeat the injury.

Clearly there are no statistics to calculate the number of us who suffer back pain at home from everyday tasks such as carrying the shopping, lifting a small child or cleaning the bath. We don't report or record it; we don't receive training for the tasks we undertake every day and we certainly don't get paid while our suffering exists. Generally, we just 'get on with it' and manage as best we can until, eventually, recovery gets us back up to speed.

The opportunities for harm are endless and yet we give little consideration to the huge number of tasks and hobbies we carry out during our time spent at home. We've all heard of the proverb, 'the straw that broke the camel's back', and sometimes that is exactly how it seems to happen. Maybe we have abused our backs with our poor posture and bad techniques for months or even years and then, one day, we casually stoop to pick up a piece of paper from the floor and it's, 'Ooh, my back!'

The striking pain is terrible. It momentarily takes your breath away and can sometimes render you unable to move for several minutes. With the muscles in spasm, from that moment on your body is screaming for relief.

For those who have not experienced such an episode, it is hard to imagine its crippling nature, and the extreme incapacity it causes may be difficult to understand. With no visible physical injury, such as a broken bone or a bleeding wound, sympathy from others can sometimes be sceptical and is often short lived. But every movement grabs like a vice. It hurts to stand, to sit, to lie down, to stay in any one position for more than a few minutes. The pain is sickening and the damage is done!

Most of us have experienced this situation and those that haven't, well, it's probably only a matter of time… Prevention, they say, is always better than cure. So what is it that subjects us all to backache?

In the 21st century, we enjoy a much more sedentary lifestyle than previous generations. Computers, television, cars and even mobile phones all contribute to behaviour which has removed the need to be constantly on the move. Communication with each other from the comfort of our homes means that our physical actions are more akin to a sudden burst of activity than a continuation of muscular suppleness.

It is a well-known fact that there are more injuries suffered in the home than anywhere else, yet there is little help or advice available to offer us protection. This book sets out to be that missing support. It offers a basic knowledge of the way our bodies work and move (chapter 2) and provides a guide to safe practice with techniques and exercises to help prevent back strain (chapters 9 to 12).

If back pain does strike, there are many suggestions, from both my knowledge and my personal experience, to help you cope and relieve the pain. I have included some important tips and helpful exercises, with illustrations, to help you prevent, recover from and reduce the risk of further injury.

It is also important to recognise when back pain is more than just a strain and when more problematic symptoms require professional medical help. In chapter 6, I describe the difference between temporary back strain and chronic back pain, as well as slipped discs.

There are many specialist organisations, therapies and treatments that are available for the treatment of back pain and its prevention. But what are the differences and what do they do? Although this book does not attempt to describe in detail the prolific number of orthodox and complementary medicines available, it sets out (chapters 13 & 14) to give a very brief history and explanation of the mainstream therapies most commonly found in both the West and other parts of the world. It also includes information about whether they are supported by a regulatory body, for which contact details are provided. Complementary medicine is a tremendous growth industry. Increasing numbers of people turn to it, some as a lifestyle choice, others seeking an effective remedy when more conventional treatments appear to have failed. Understanding what it can offer and what the choices are – and the limitations – can help anyone with a back problem focus on what will be right for them.

Running a home is one of the most demanding occupations. We need to be cooks, cleaners, organisers, financial experts, gardeners, drivers – the list goes on and on. All of these tasks become more difficult, if not impossible, with a bad back. Just lifting a kettle to make a cup of tea can put strain on those painful muscles. But apart from the physical suffering of back pain, another, more subtle crippling and underestimated effect of long-term disability can be that of isolation and depression. Avoiding such a downward spiral requires a pro-active approach right from the outset. I talk about this in chapter 7.

With such a high incidence of back pain, mostly due to our modern, sedentary lifestyle, the odds are clearly stacked against us. This book therefore aims to provide a comprehensive guide to understanding the common causes of low back pain and how to manage this painful condition. I offer many practical techniques relevant to common, everyday activities both within the home and during leisure time, in order both to evade the development of back pain and to prevent its recurrence.

Key points

- Back pain in the UK is claimed to be the next most common ailment to the common cold.

- Government legislation exists to protect workers, but there is no help or advice available for those at home.

- There are more injuries in the home than anywhere else.

Chapter 2

How we walk on two legs

Evolution has enabled us to walk upright, supported by our spinal bones. If, as some say, prehistoric man once walked on all fours, over many thousands of years we have adapted and developed the human frame to give us the freedom to stand upright and use our hands and arms for other, more intricate, tasks.

To appreciate why our backs can give us problems, especially to cause us pain and restrictive movement, it is helpful to understand how this part of our skeletal frame works and the many functions it has to perform. Caring for our spines both mechanically and nutritionally is vital to our general health. It is, after all, one of the most important parts of our body and its knobbly structure is far more than a scaffold tower on which to place the head.

The structures and systems that give us mobility and strength can never work in isolation. Just as with any sporting or business team, each component relies on the support of the others for its effectiveness. Bones, muscles and other soft tissues combine to work together. However, any one part can be injured and cause pain if subjected to repetitive or excessive strain, such as a sudden unplanned movement, twisting or distorted alignment. If you want to take care of your own back, it is a good idea, therefore, to have a basic understanding of the way backs work.

Viewed from the side, the spine looks like an elongated 'S' shape (see Figure 2.1). It is designed both to carry and to make allowance for the space required for most of our vital organs as well as balancing our weight so that we do not tip over.

The spinal column is made up of 33 irregularly shaped, ring-like small

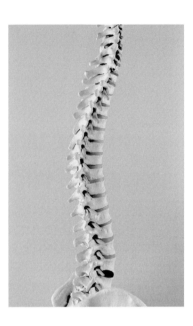

Figure 2.1 Side view of the spinal column showing the normal elongated 'S' shape.

bones. Together these act like a continuous tube in which to encase and protect our spinal cord, which is the continuation of the brain and extends from the head downwards. These 33 bones are classified into three main sections.

The top seven vertebrae form the smaller cervical bones, which curve slightly inwards to make the neck. The next 12 vertebrae, called the thoracic segment, curve slightly outwards. It is to these bones that the ribs are attached and this forms a protective enclosure for the lungs and heart.

The lower segment, the lumbar spine, is the area most at risk of injury. It contains five, or in some cases six, vertebrae, again curving slightly inwards. These are rather larger than the higher bones as they are not only responsible for supporting the main abdominal organs, but also transmit most of the upper body's weight. The shapes of these individual vertebrae differ a little but generally comprise a hollow ring with a bony 'process' protruding, to which the muscles are attached.

The last nine bones of the spinal column are fused together into two larger bones. The sacrum is formed by five united vertebrae and finally, the coccyx is made up of a further four small bones bonded together.

To prevent the vertebrae scraping against each other in movement, flat round cushions called 'intervertebral discs' are situated between each of the bones. These act as 'shock absorbers' and allow a limited amount of movement between each of the vertebrae so that we can bend, twist and adjust our position to maintain our balance. These discs have the appearance of a hard outer covering with a jelly-like centre, called the nucleus. They can be squashed down and change shape under pressure. There is no blood supply to the discs – they have to get their oxygen and nutrients from the movement of the spine. Therefore, the more movement, the healthier and firmer the discs will be.

These intervertebral discs, although capable of withstanding enormous forces, are also frequently at risk of injury. An accident, wear and tear or excessive pressure when lifting awkwardly, can lead to the outer covering of the disc rupturing, causing the inner material to bulge out or become prolapsed see Figure 2.2. This can cause pressure to be placed on the nerve which leaves the spinal column at that level. The result can be extremely painful, putting the muscle into spasm and causing stiffness, or perhaps even numbness, to the part of the body which is supplied by that particular nerve. Unlike most other tissues in the body, damaged intervertebral discs are very slow to heal since, as previously mentioned, they have no blood supply of their own. This is one of the common reasons why back injuries take so long to recover.

It is also a known fact that you grow taller while you're asleep in bed – yes really! At night, when you lie down and pressure is taken off the spine, water is drawn into the jelly-like centre of the discs and the nucleus swells up again.

Figure 2.2 Frontal view of the spinal column showing a prolapsed intervertebral disc.

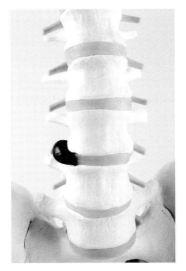

By the morning, you are ever so slightly taller than you were the night before. However, during the day, normal movement and activity restore the length of the spinal column to its original height.

The spinal cord, which runs from the head down through the centre of each of the spinal bones, is made up of millions of tiny nerve fibres. To further protect the cord from its bony casing, a colourless liquid, called the spinal fluid, surrounds these nerve fibres. This is held within a protective membrane called the *dura mater*. It acts rather like a waterproof sack.

As the spinal cord descends through the centre of the spinal bones, 31 pairs of nerve roots exit the spine, one pair between each of the vertebrae. These carry messages (electrical impulses) to and from the brain, to signal voluntary and involuntary movement and sensation specific to the area of the body supplied by each nerve. It is these nerves that allow you to control your muscles, perceive touch, pain and temperature, as well as manage bladder and bowel movement.

We have all experienced numbness or tingling sensations when a nerve has been squashed and its normal passage of electrical impulses has been temporarily interrupted. An example of this 'pins and needles' sensation can sometimes be felt after kneeling and resting back on our heels for a long period of time. When you stand up and the pressure is once again released, the feeling of hundreds of tiny pin-pricks dancing beneath the skin demonstrates the return of nerves and circulation to the area.

Down the length of the spine, you can feel a series of bony lumps. These are part of the vertebrae and are called the 'spinous' and 'transverse' processes, to which the muscles are attached by tendons.

Each individual spinal joint does not have a wide range of movement, but collectively they allow us great flexibility, so that we can arch a limited distance backwards, bend a long way forwards and twist or lean from side to side. It is the irregularity of the shapes of the vertebrae that dictate that we can bend further forwards than backwards. The top seven bones, the cervical segment, being smaller, are able to give us the greatest amount of flexibility so that we can turn and tip our head in many directions with ease.

So what gives us our strength? There is a huge network of muscles involved in body movement; these muscles represent what we know as the body's flesh. Arranged in criss-crossing intricate layers, their job is to pull the bones to which they are attached. From tiny subtle movements to taking vigorous exercise, we are able to control each decisive action with well-defined accuracy. The average human body contains a total of approximately 640 muscles; these make up about two-fifths of a male's weight. Although the female form contains the same number, they account for a slightly smaller proportion of overall weight.

As you can feel when you run your hand down your back, there are no muscles crossing over the backbone. However, a thick bundle of muscle fibres and tendons runs more or less vertically in the groove alongside the spine and connects to each one of the vertebrae. Imagine a thick, tight band of muscle fibres fixed at the bottom, which divides into two and gradually fans out on either side, reaching up towards the shoulder blades. At its lower portion, the concentration of muscle in the lumber region is where most of the strain is absorbed.

Difficult, and some might say, perplexing names relate to each of the muscles, but generally their titles reflect either their shape, their position or the corresponding bone to which they are attached. Although it is not necessary to remember such medical terminology, as an example, the three long, thin striated muscles which are responsible for elevating and straightening our spines are called the *Erector Spinae*. Their main responsibility is to extend the spine and maintain our correct curvature, and it is these muscles which often suffer strain as we carry out our daily activities.

The *Erector Spinae* muscles are small in size compared to the two larger muscles, which spread like huge, flat triangles up towards the shoulders and across the broadest part on either side of our back and chest wall. These particular muscles are responsible for extending, rotating and lowering our arms as well as pulling our shoulders back. Although these muscles cover the largest surface area of any of the body's muscles, they do not have the density and strength of, say, the thigh muscles.

When considering our human strength, we may perhaps think of our backs as the main 'power-house', but it is actually our thigh and abdominal muscles that are most capable of supporting our body when moving heavy objects or undertaking strain of some kind. If the supporting muscle groups, in particular the abdominal muscles, are not used to best effect, then it is the back muscles which are left to take most of the strain unaided and it is this that renders us most at risk of injury.

To test the effectiveness of your abdominal muscles, stand upright with your feet shoulder-width apart, your bottom tucked in and lean slightly backwards. In this position you should be able to feel your abdominal muscles tightening slightly in order to support you. Similarly, whilst looking forwards and with a straight back, if you bend slightly at the knees, you will again feel a slight tension across the abdomen. Another source of strength, which is often ignored, are the gluteus or buttock muscles. By clenching these muscles, the abdominal muscles are almost automatically brought into action. It is this support that is so important both in exercises to strengthen back muscles and in carrying out everyday tasks.

Muscles are only able to pull and relax. They cannot push. This means that no one muscle can work in isolation; they have to work in pairs. As one muscle tightens and contracts, its opposite partner relaxes, allowing the movement. Reversing the actions of both muscles restores the original position.

From the description I've given of the way our bones and muscles work, you could be forgiven for thinking that we ought to be super-powerful, designed and built to take on any heavy task we choose. Repetitive stress or pressure on the lower region of our back, however, will eventually send out its own warning – pain! Just like an over-stretched elastic band, excessive strain can eventually diminish the ability of the muscles to maintain their elasticity, causing pain and loss of strength. Considering the amount of weight that is already bearing down onto the lumbar region, any more additional strain can compress the vertebrae together, causing low back pain and injury.

Almost all of our household chores involve leaning forwards. We generally allow our backs to take the strain, whether it is cleaning the bath, making the bed, sweeping the floor, carrying the shopping or cleaning the car. The list is endless. In our busy daily lives we pay little attention to the constant wear and tear we consistently impose on our back muscles.

Help is at hand, however, if we are prepared to use it. The strength and effect of our abdominal muscles should not be underestimated in their ability to support the lower back. This group of muscles runs in layers vertically and diagonally across the abdomen and not only supports the abdominal organs, but together with the muscles of the back and buttocks, is able to encourage good alignment of the spine and posture.

Much is written and stated about posture and its importance in relation to the health of our spines. Although a bad back will not be cured by good posture alone, its influence on the back's recovery and on the prevention of future problems should not be undervalued. Our increasingly sedentary lifestyle, with or without the perhaps excess weight accumulated around the girdle, means these important muscle groups have to work very hard just to maintain good mobility and flexibility.

Factors that increase the risk of back problems

'Lordosis' is a common problem. This is the exaggerated curve of the spine projecting the buttocks, accompanied very often by a large protruding stomach. It can leave the lower lumbar region very vulnerable to weakness as it grossly distorts the correct alignment of the spine.

Many tall individuals suffer with back pain due to poor posture, especially with the need for persistent stooping and the extra exertion required for lifting and bending. As across the world our peoples are gradually becoming taller in stature, we are slow to respond to the need to accommodate those whose height is above 1.9 metres and for whom the standard height of everyday appliances, worktops and equipment is now too low.

Pregnancy will obviously stretch the abdominal muscles to extreme as well as putting excessive weight and drag on the lower back. Many expectant women understandably experience constant low back pain. This is because during the last two trimesters of pregnancy, the fetus can increase the curvature of the mother's spine by its pressure. Now that new mothers are in hospital for such a short time after the delivery of their babies, the times when physiotherapists routinely visited post-natal wards have sadly gone. It is necessary, however, that effective postnatal exercises are practised at home in order to restore the over-worked muscles back to their original status, although for many of us the firm, flat tummy is never quite as strong as before.

The processes of aging also affect our spinal tissues. With increasing age, the intervertebral discs lose some of the pressure held within them, causing them to bulge slightly like a flat tyre. They can become stiffer and therefore more vulnerable to injury. With the advancing years, bone mineral is also lost from the vertebrae. This is especially noticeable in post-menopausal women; combined with the loss of pressure in the discs, this can lead to a loss in height. This, however, does not mean that back pain is an inevitable part of ageing.

Physical exercise, as we know, strengthens muscles. It is also known that physically active people have both stronger discs and vertebrae, whereas persistent lack of use and general inactivity weaken them. This is true for the elderly as well as the young. We do need to be aware, however, that spontaneous or ill-prepared physical activity by those not generally very active, such as gardening on the first good day of spring, will dramatically increase the risk of back injury.

Key points

- Thirty-three irregularly shaped bones make up the spinal column.

- Flat, round cushions called intervertebral discs act as shock absorbers between the spinal bones.

- The muscles attached to the lumbar spinal bones are the most likely to suffer strain.

- The abdominal, buttock and thigh muscles provide essential support for the back muscles.

- Good posture is essential to successful back care.

- Physical exercise strengthens both muscles and vertebrae, whereas inactivity weakens them.

- Back pain is not an inevitable part of ageing

Chapter 3

Nutrition and its benefits

No programme for improved health and fitness can ever be attempted in isolation from the value of good nutrition. The importance of both developing and maintaining a healthy body is crucial when our mobility and independence are at stake.

Unfortunately, there are no magical nutritional 'cures' for back ache. Prevention, however, is always better than cure and a diet which contains all the necessary proteins and vitamins for healthy bones and muscles will go a long way towards helping to prevent the development of back problems in the first place. A combination of health-giving foods and exercise will also aid recovery from back pain by providing improved fitness and energy.

For many of us, one of the greatest obstacles to relieving that nagging back ache is the problem of obesity. The added weight placed upon the lower back can distort the correct alignment of the spine. This not only causes fatigue, but, more seriously, places uneven pressure on the vertebrae and increases the risk of a slipped disc.

Losing weight is not easy. Dieticians recommend that following a balanced, healthy-eating diet, combined with exercise, is by far the best way to reduce excessive weight, even though progress may appear to be slow. Crash diets, and there are very many different programmes available, can sometimes result in nutritional imbalance. As well as making you feel unwell and unnecessarily exhausted from sudden weight loss, your general health may also be compromised. It is therefore important to ensure a sensible and nutritious approach to eating.

Strong muscles rely to a great extent upon a diet containing 10-15% protein. It is not just athletes who need to eat protein, such as meat, fish, cheese, milk and eggs to help build strong muscles. We may not be planning to run a marathon, but running a home can be just as exhausting!

Fresh fruit, vegetables and protein will also help reduce the body's susceptibility to infection, as well as other illnesses and some degenerative diseases. The World Health Organisation recommends five portions of fruit and vegetables a day. This may sound a lot, but including one piece of fruit with each meal, together with the vegetables or salad with your main meal, should make this reasonably easy to achieve.

Vitamins and minerals for bones and joints

One of the major discoveries of the 20th century was that of vitamins and the importance these nutrients have as the basis for a healthy diet. The most important vitamins needed for bone formation are vitamins A, C and D. Trace minerals are also important and include fluorine, calcium, copper, phosphorus and magnesium. The minute amounts required of these minerals, and delicate balance between deficiency and toxicity, are best managed by including a wide variety of fresh fruit and vegetables.

Calcium
Calcium is a particularly vital component of our bones and teeth. It is also needed for the smooth functioning of nerves and muscles. Foods rich in calcium are milk, cheese, sardines (including the bones), dark green leafy vegetables and sesame seeds. With age, however, more calcium is lost from our bones than is replaced. Osteoporosis, or brittle bone disease as it is sometimes called, results from the loss of calcium and bone density. This painful condition, which is particularly prevalent in post-menopausal women, can cause the spinal column to become weak and compressed, resulting in loss of height and sometimes a stooped posture. Preventative measures, such as regular weight-bearing exercise – walking or jogging – will help maintain the density of bones and can help to reduce vital mineral loss.

Vitamin D

Vitamin D is sometimes referred to as the 'sunshine' vitamin, since it is made by our bodies in response to sunlight as well as being absorbed from certain foods. It is responsible for our bodies taking in calcium and phosphorus, which are both vital for bone, muscle and nerve growth. Even in some countries of the northern hemisphere it is thought that enough vitamin D can be absorbed during the summer months to be sufficient for the year. However, for people who spend most of their time indoors, such as those with limited mobility, there is considerable risk of deficiency of this valuable vitamin without sufficient dietary intake.

Deficiency of vitamin D is known to cause rickets in children, (a softening and irregular growth of the bones resulting in deformity) and osteomalacia, which is the adult form of rickets, causing much pain and increasing the likelihood of fractures. Such is the importance of vitamin D that in some western countries, including the United Kingdom, some fortified foods such as margarine and breakfast cereals are required by law to contain it.

Vitamin D, which is a fat-soluble compound, is converted in the kidneys and acts like a hormone to control and regulate the level of calcium in the bones. Although it is synthesised in the skin and can be stored for a long period of time in the body, a small regular dietary consumption is also a good idea. Good sources of vitamin D are liver and oily fish, such as sardines, mackerel and salmon. The value of these foods cannot be underestimated since the fatty acids within the fish can also help to suppress inflammation and, in doing so, help reduce pain in the joints. And you do not need to eat bucket-loads either, as just a 100 gram serving twice a week will provide you with the recommended weekly intake.

Vitamin C

Vitamin C, or ascorbic acid as it is also known, is another essential vitamin responsible for the development and maintenance of strong bones, collagen (a protein constituent of fibrous tissue), cartilage and nerves. Although renowned for its use in combating colds and other infectious diseases, it also helps to produce noradrenaline, the hormone which regulates blood flow. Oxygen carried in the blood is essential for our muscles in order to function well. It is often the lack of oxygen to muscle fibres that causes strains to occur when they are put under stress.

Our bodies cannot manufacture most vitamins, so vital nutrients, like vitamin

C, have to be absorbed by eating the foods which contain them. Vitamin C is water soluble and cannot be stored in the body, so frequent intake through diet is essential for good health.

The normal adult requirement of vitamin C is 40 milligrams a day. Although this sounds a lot, it can be provided by just one portion of fruit or vegetables. Fortunately, vitamin C is contained in varying amounts in some of our most common and easily available foods. Some of the highest concentrations are found in citrus fruits such as oranges, lemons and grapefruit, but kale and other dark green vegetables also contain large amounts of this valuable vitamin. In fact most root and green vegetables, such as potatoes, cabbage and broccoli also contain vitamin C, as do strawberries, blackcurrants, guavas, kiwi fruit and peppers.

Vitamin supplements and factors affecting vitamin requirements

Some manufacturers of breakfast cereals also include many vitamin supplements in their products, often to the value of 30-40% of the recommended daily intake. Vitamin D is included in some, too.

It is important that smokers are aware that they require double the daily amount of vitamins compared with non-smokers. Smoking causes the spinal discs to age faster than normal and to stiffen up. This inhibits the blood supply and oxygen from enriching the intervertebral discs, which can significantly increase the risk of a disc becoming displaced.

Nutritional supplements

Nutritional supplements are widely available and indeed are enthusiastically advertised for all sorts of medical conditions, including back and joint pain. For this problem, glucosamine sulphate and chondroiton sulphate supplements are believed to improve the repair and formation of cartilage in inflamed joints as well as providing pain relief. However, it should be pointed out that these supplements are predominately recommended to aid relief in osteoarthritis rather than simple back pain, where muscular strain is generally the main problem.

Numerous studies over recent years would appear to provide some evidence that pain can indeed be reduced by the use of these supplements. If you are already taking other analgesic medication and wish to try one of these products, it is strongly recommended that the advice of a medical practitioner is sought before taking additional compounds since combining orthodox medication with nutritional supplements may be detrimental to your health.

Remember, a well-balanced diet should really provide all the protein, vitamins and minerals necessary for good bone formation, and the repair of muscles and nerves.

Caffeine – cutting down

Reducing the amount of caffeine can also be helpful to the health of your back. Caffeine, which is a mild stimulant, can narrow the tiny blood vessels at the tips of the smaller arteries. Spinal tendons, which rely on an adequate blood supply to provide both oxygen and nutrients, can be compromised and this can also delay healing. Furthermore, excessive intake of caffeine can accelerate the loss of calcium and minerals from the bone.

If coffee, which carries the highest proportion of caffeine, is a frequent and regular daytime drink for you, you might wish to change to the decaffeinated alternative. Ground coffee contains almost twice as much as instant. Other sources of caffeine include dark chocolate, tea and cola. There are lesser amounts in cocoa, milk chocolate and drinking chocolate.

Having said this, it is not advisable to dramatically reduce your consumption of caffeine or cut it out altogether in one fell swoop, as the sudden withdrawal can cause headaches and lethargy. Both of these symptoms are miserable and will make you far less inclined to want to exercise. Therefore, if you feel your usual intake is, perhaps, more than it should be, reduce it slowly over a week or two.

Some of the pain killers on the market have caffeine as one of their ingredients. This is because paradoxically, caffeine enhances the analgesic effect of other pain killers, like paracetamol.

Antioxidants

A diet which is low in antioxidants, particularly the trace mineral selenium, may predispose some people to joint problems. Kale is an excellent source of two of the antioxidants – vitamin A and beta carotene. Of all the vegetables, kale is one of the richest sources of calcium, which is essential for healthy bones. It also contains iron and folate (folic acid), which is a constituent of the vitamin B complex.

Water and keeping hydrated

Water is the least appreciated but one of the most important factors when considering nutrition in relation to back care. Throughout life our bodies must be well hydrated. It is well known that water is essential for the maintenance of all our major organs, circulation and brain. Since the distribution of water in our bodies is prioritised to these vital areas, sometimes an insufficient water intake can mean that some parts, in particular the intervertebral discs, receive less than they need. The discs, which are made up of a gel-like substance encased within a tough, pliable covering, are mostly made up of water. Acting as shock absorbers between each of the spinal bones, water is slowly squeezed out of the discs throughout the day, to be mostly re-hydrated again while we sleep at night. During the daytime it is activity such as moving the spine back and forth in exercise that allows any extra water available to be reabsorbed into the discs.

It is easy to see how dehydration may affect the pressure within the discs, so that the outer casing loses its uniformity and becomes distorted. This can affect the ability of the discs to support the upper body efficiently and may result in pain and, in extreme cases, even a prolapsed disc. Stiffness on moving, particularly when bending or straightening, is often the first sign that the discs have become dehydrated and less stable. As they become squeezed and out of alignment, they can eventually press on the sciatic nerve, causing intense pain down the back of the leg. It is also worth noting that a damaged disc is less able to reabsorb fluid, which can lead to a prolonged recovery.

In conclusion...

It is clear that good nutrition plays a very important part in the health of our bones, muscles and nerves. Recovery from back pain and our ability to strengthen the structures which have been injured rely to a great extent upon the regeneration of cells to replace those which have been damaged. This depends on a well-balanced diet which contains all the necessary nutrients.

Key points

- Good nutrition, in the form of protein and vitamins for healthy bones and muscles, will help prevent back problems and aid recovery from back pain.

- Obesity places strain on the lower back, distorting the correct alignment of the spine.

- Vitamins A, C and D are essential for good bone growth.

- Calcium is a vital component of our bones and teeth.

- Vitamin D can help to suppress inflammation and reduce pain in joints.

- Vitamin C is essential for strong bones, cartilage and nerves.

- Smoking causes the spinal discs to age faster and stiffen up.

- Supplements, such as glucosamine and chondroitin, may be helpful in reducing inflammation but are intended for sufferers of osteo-arthritis rather than simple back pain caused by muscle strain or sprain.

- An excessive intake of caffeine can accelerate the loss of calcium from bones.

Chapter 4

Myths and misconceptions

Back pain, as the statistics demonstrate, is extremely common. In the same way that everybody has a view and advice to give on the best way to cope with and eliminate the symptoms of a head cold, personal experiences of back pain also bring forth theories and guidance without necessarily the professional knowledge to support it. From this inevitably grow myths and misconceptions which, although given with good intention, give rise to a great deal of conflicting information and confusion.

There is also much evidence to suggest that the way in which we overwork our spines and the connecting muscles can do us a great deal of harm. Add this to the many misunderstandings about back care and we not only inhibit our ability to recover speedily from injury, but can also subject ourselves to unnecessary weakening of our back muscles. How to assess the risk involved in a manual task and carry it out safely is more fully discussed in chapter 8; here I will tackle the most common misunderstandings about what is good and bad for backs.

'Put your back into it'

Seldom do the sayings and proverbs of past generations convey anything but good sound advice but one such phrase, 'Put your back into it', can certainly be misinterpreted. This saying might suggest that increasing physical effort by using enormous force to push, pull or lift something, will help the desired task to be better achieved. It is more likely, however, to have the opposite effect and even give you an injury. Its inference, that the spine is always the strongest part of the body, sometimes leads us to undertake physical effort far beyond our safe capability.

'You should sleep on a hard mattress'

How often have we been enticed to purchase an extra firm 'orthopaedic' mattress, believing it to be good for our backs? A mattress that is too hard and does not yield slightly to the contours of our spine can put considerable strain on that small area in the lower lumbar region which is left with no base on which to rest. The back muscles, when they should be completely relaxed, are therefore given the work of supporting the weight of the lower organs of the body throughout the night. This can result in stiffness and pain in the mornings. A slightly gentler mattress, therefore, will not only provide consistent support along the length of the natural curvature of the spine, but will aid more restful sleep.

It is important when buying a mattress to take plenty of time to try it out for comfort before making your choice. Lie on the bed. All good stores provide shoe protection on their display beds. Mattresses should be neither too hard nor too soft. Slide a hand under the small of your back and feel if there is a gap. Lie on your side or in the position which you normally find most comfortable at night to establish whether the whole line of your body is straight and will be adequately supported during the hours of rest and sleep. A mattress which sags is equally bad for you. Spending many hours curved like the shape of a slice of melon will mean that you will not only start the next day with a stiff, aching back but with lethargy as well from insufficient quality sleep.

It is a very good idea to try a range of beds from different manufacturers before making your choice. A bed should be one of our most important purchases, especially as we spend almost one third of our lives in bed, so don't be afraid to be fussy. You will be spending many hours of every day either appreciating or regretting your eventual choice.

'I hurt my back because I got tired'

One fact which often causes surprise is the time of day when you are most likely to strain your back. It is not always in the late evening when you are tired, but more likely to be in the early morning before the muscles have had time to warm up. The pain, however, may not be felt until later in the day or even when you eventually sit down to rest. Unfortunately, before embarking on household tasks or 'DIY' jobs, we seldom consider that we should 'warm up' our muscles like a sportsman. It may seem a little extreme to be stretching and carrying out a few exercises before hanging wallpaper or digging the garden, but it can be the difference between a successful day and one which results in misery.

'I've put my back out'

Another misconception is that a sudden, severe onset of back pain is always as the result of a 'slipped disc'. Intervertebral discs do not just carelessly slip out of position and in fact less than 5% of all back pain suffered is the result of a disc becoming displaced or squeezed between the bones of the spine. The vast majority of back pain is caused by the distressing spasm resulting from over-stretched muscles.

However, if the symptoms appear more serious than just muscle spasm with generalised aching, and involve leg pain, severe immobility or numbness/pins and needles down the legs, then the possibility of a prolapsed disc should be considered. This should be examined by a medical practitioner as the situation requires accurate diagnosis before embarking on any programme of rehabilitation. Very occasionally, as the result of severe trauma such as a fall or sporting injury, a fracture dislocation is possible, but this is a matter requiring urgent medical attention.

'I need to lie on the floor for six weeks'

At one time, when back pain struck, it was common practice to lie on the floor for perhaps up to six weeks, or to go to bed and stay there until the pain subsided. Although initially rest and analgesics (pain-killers) for a day or two will help to relax the injured muscles and relieve spasm, prolonged bed rest has now been proven to worsen the pain and delay recovery. Walking and gentle exercise should be resumed as soon as they can be tolerated. If the spasm is so bad that walking is too painful, frequent stretching and rotation of your ankles will help to stimulate the circulation to your legs and lower part of your body.

'I'm too young to get back ache'

A popular misconception held by young and fit individuals is that they cannot harm their backs because they are supple and their muscles well developed. Although youth and fitness are of enormous benefit, nobody can be said to be exempt from a back injury. A single movement repetitively carried out, such as stooping to polish a car, or maintaining an awkward position, for example, sitting slumped in a chair, can bring about the first signs of weakness.

Contrary to common belief, back pain is not infrequent in 30-50 year olds. This is often a time when poor posture and inappropriate lifting techniques which have persisted during the earlier years eventually reveal a physical weakness in the back muscles. Good practice learned in childhood is the best protection against harm. In later years, although natural degenerative processes are responsible for a slight shortening of the spine, reduced muscle tone and decreased bone strength and thickness, elderly people are less likely to over-estimate their ability to move or lift a heavy item. Young men in particular are often reluctant to ask for assistance with a heavy load, perhaps fearing that to do so may appear weak in the presence of their peers.

'I hurt my back once, so I know it is weak'

Back problems developed in youth or middle age do not have to be an indication that it is the start of a slippery downhill slide into a world of disability, walking sticks or wheelchairs. Strengthening exercises, improved posture and more accurately assessing the tasks to be carried out, will help to prevent recurrence.

'If I ignore it, it will go away'

Back pain is not something in your imagination or which can easily be 'worked off' by persevering with a strenuous physical task. All pain is real and a symptom that something is wrong. Ignoring the pain and continuing with the activity in the hope that eventually it will go away, will more likely exacerbate the problem and delay healing of the strained tissues.

'An operation is the only answer'

Unfortunately there is no 'quick fix' for back pain. Surgery to the back does not guarantee to cure all types of back pain in the long term. Statistics show that up to 30% of patients may suffer in some way from the effects of the surgery or may not even gain adequate relief from their original back ache. Your orthopaedic surgeon will discuss both the need and implications of any kind of invasive procedure to make sure that you fully understand the anticipated outcome of such surgery. He will also want to be sure that all other more conservative treatments have been thoroughly explored first.

'You can see that I am in pain'

There are very few signs, if any, to the casual observer that someone is suffering from constant, nagging back pain. Recovering from back pain can take anything from a few days to several weeks. This sometimes means that sympathy and patience can wear a little thin, even drawing accusations of laziness or being 'work-shy'. Back pain is not, however, a problem that you have to live with. There are many solutions, appropriate to individual circumstances, including both orthodox medical treatments and alternative therapies, which can be very helpful.

Positive conclusion

Back pain that is not actively challenged is unlikely to be a 'once-in-a-lifetime' event. It is important to keep that in mind – it is not a myth! However, when life is back to normal and full mobility restored, the whole event and its accompanying misery may be quickly forgotten. Do not drop your guard – it is a recognised fact that following one episode of back pain, you are three to four times more likely to suffer its wrath again. Therefore, as soon as full mobility has been restored is the time to make the conscious decision to improve your everyday posture and lifting techniques. This makes muscle-strengthening exercises (see chapter 12) all the more important to prevent that recurrence. First, however, we will look at the causes of back pain.

Key points

- Your spine needs the support of many of your body's muscles and is not the strongest part of your body.

- Sleep on a bed that is soft enough to let your spine rest in its natural 'S' shape, but firm enough to support its length.

- Warm up your back muscles before using them for anything stenuous – when you wake in the morning they will have stiffened up.

- Look after your back whatever age you are – relatively young people get back problems and store up trouble for the future through bad habits.

- Most (95%) of back pain results from overstretched muscles – less than 5% from a 'slipped disc'.

- Surgical procedures are necessary only for a very few people.

- Keeping mobile is the best way to help your back recover...

- ... but do not persist with any activity that is clearly making the pain worse

- Just because you have had a problem in the past does not mean you will again – future trouble can be avoided, especially if you take the preventive measures in this book!

Chapter 5

Everyday causes of back pain

There are literally hundreds of ways in which you can strain your back whilst carrying out everyday household and leisure activities.

Statistics show that men and women suffer back pain in about the same proportions. Not so long ago it used to be that many men suffered mostly from the effects of heavy and repetitive lifting. Back pain in women was often the result of a variety of monotonous tasks such as cleaning, or standing for long periods of time in either factories or shops. Today, men are just as likely to suffer from the effects of sedentary occupations and women are more frequently undertaking many of the more manual occupations. For both sexes, juggling the complexities of managing a job with running a home can cause emotional tension, which is not only detrimental to general health but can increase stress in the performance of physical activities.

It is beyond the scope of this book to illustrate more than a few of the most common causes of back pain likely to occur both in the home or during our time spent away from work, but the general principles can be applied to most of our actions. Here are a few suggestions which you may find helpful in the prevention of back strain. They are listed alphabetically for ease of location, not in order of risk.

Beds

We spend as much as one third of our lives lying in bed. In order to sleep well, the bed must be comfortable and our position relaxed and well supported. It is whilst sleeping that much of the healing and vital cell replacement is carried out by our bodies.

Tips

- Try not to lie prone (face down) in bed as the arch in your spine is increased beyond its normal curvature. It is better to lie on your side or back.
- If lying on your side is uncomfortable, try placing a pillow between your knees so that your pelvis and lower back are kept aligned.
- Be aware that if you lie on your side with your shoulders raised by your pillow, this is inclined to twist the natural alignment of your body as well as place strain on your neck muscles.
- If you prefer lying on your back, a pillow placed beneath your knees can help reduce the curvature of your spine so that support is improved throughout its length.
- Position your head pillow so that it supports your head and neck only. Pressing the pillow into the curvature of your neck may also improve comfort.

Car seats

Depending on the make and model of the vehicle, car seats are manufactured to a standard design. Unfortunately, we do not all comfortably conform to the contours of the seats because our individual shapes and heights differ slightly. The lengths of our spines vary according to our general physique. This means that the support offered by any car seat to our lower backs may not always be in the correct position. On a long journey, when a driver may sit for a prolonged period of time in a fixed and specific pose, back strain is inevitable. Not only do our back muscles suffer if our seated position is slumped, but for some women in particular, who often tend to lift their feet off the floor to operate the pedals, this strain is exaggerated.

Tips

- When seated, your knees should ideally be the same height or slightly higher than your hips. Test the strain placed on your lower back by simulating an 'emergency stop' to ensure your position is comfortable.

- Position the seat close enough to the steering wheel to enable you to reach the pedals with comfort and bring the back of the seat into an almost upright position to support the curve of your back.
- If it helps, use a small cushion or piece of foam to fit snugly into the lower lumbar area of your back. This not only helps to correct the alignment of your spine, but will act as a brace for your back if both your feet are elevated simultaneously, as in an emergency stop.
- On a lengthy journey, make it a policy to allow time for breaks. Stop every 1-2 hours and walk about to stretch both your leg and back muscles. Your alertness will also be improved by this practice.

Caring for others in the home

The safest and most natural way to carry a newborn baby is to cradle it in both arms close to your body. Not only is the baby secure but is held close to the holder's centre of gravity. As the child develops and gets heavier, however, convenience often dictates that the toddler is sat astride one hip, supported by just one arm. In order to counter-balance the weight, the hip is tilted and the parent/carer's body is leaned away from the additional weight, creating a distorted sideways 'S' shape. A basket of washing supported by one hip is another example of this method of carrying (see Fig. 5.1). Yes, we've all done it and despite its potential danger, it must be accepted that such a practice is unlikely to change. The necessity for improved muscular tone and strength in the lower back is therefore imperative.

It is not just those caring for young children who are at risk. There are thousands of people, both male and female, who have the responsibility of caring for a sick, disabled or elderly relative in their home. Despite the variety of equipment and gadgets accessible on the market, as well as, for some, the availability of professional carers to assist with daily living activities, it still falls to family members to manage most of the care.

Frequent making of beds that are too low, help with dressing, bathing and toileting, extra shopping, cleaning and laundry are just a very few of the additional strains placed on your lower back. Add to this the permanent state of tiredness that exists from, perhaps, interrupted sleep, and the demands on your body are enormous.

Figure 5.1 Distorted sideways 'S' shape – see how carrying a weight on your hip can affect your posture.

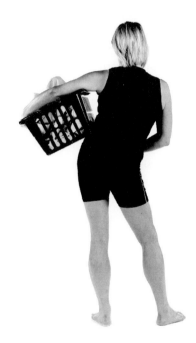

An object or weight that you need to lift will usually be one of two kinds: stable or unstable. A stable weight is generally a solid object with a clearly defined shape, which can be managed according to its weight and size. On the other hand, carrying a small child or assisting an adult can be far more hazardous. It is the unexpected strain, for which you have no protection, that can inflict an instant and intolerable snatch on your back muscles.

Small children can have a tendency spontaneously to throw their weight away from your centre of gravity whilst being carried. A sick or elderly person, having lost their confidence and strength, may hang onto or grab the arm of a chair or handrail when you are helping to mobilise them, just when you least expect it. The resulting wrench can be catastrophic to your own balance and muscles.

Tips

- Be aware of the strain on your back when carrying a small child on your hip. Try to keep an upright posture and change sides frequently to avoid a persistent strain to the muscles on one side.
- If you are responsible for looking after an elderly or disabled relative, take

the time to write a list of all the physically taxing tasks that need to be done on a regular basis and which put your back muscles under most strain.

- Look at each task individually to see whether anything can be done to make your life easier. For example, would transfers onto and off the bed and bed-making be easier if the bed was raised on blocks to make it higher? Can furniture be rearranged in a room to give you more space in which to manoeuvre? Can the daily routine be changed so that heavier tasks can be done when other family members are present?

Cooking

Cooking may seem to be an activity unlikely to cause back pain, but low-level ovens, particularly, can be extremely hazardous. Great care needs to be taken when inserting and withdrawing fully laden large roasting tins, glass casseroles or other cookware, especially if they contain liquid or piping hot food. Add to this the physical manoeuvre of bending, lifting and sometimes, turning, and back muscle spasm at this time can be catastrophic! Beware, too, of peering into a glass-fronted oven door to assess the baking progress with a stooping posture when your thoughts are more concerned with the contents of the oven than the straightness of your back.

Tips

- Always use a good quality, heat-resistant oven glove so that your movements do not need to be rushed.
- Approach the opened oven with one foot in front of the other and bend at the knees. This will aid your balance.
- Use your thigh muscles to push you up into a standing position before turning away from the cooker.
- Keep your back straight at all times.

Falling

The jarring from a fall is another likely cause of back pain. It may seem unlikely that such an injury will occur in your own home or garden, but accidents of this kind are common-place. Some might say that most are avoidable, but that doesn't mean they don't happen. Slipping on a wet kitchen or bathroom floor; tripping over an uneven carpet, toys or shoes; falling from a chair whilst changing a light bulb; or slipping in the shower or bath – the potential hazards are numerous.

Tips

- Try as far as you can to assess the risk of the task you intend to carry out. You may have done it hundreds of times and got away without it causing harm to you, but was that luck and could it run out?
- Take just a moment to consider your environment to reduce the risk – it's worth it (see chapter 8).

Gardening

Gardening, of course, is another very common cause of back pain. The sudden appearance of spring with the first warm, dry day and we're out there digging the soil, cutting the grass and clearing up the debris that the winter months have claimed. Full of enthusiasm, we stoop, twist, lift and generally put our backs through a range of tortuous movements that we are ill prepared for. The very action of digging with a spade or fork, especially in heavy or clay soil, requires twisting at the same time as lifting and is a movement that is likely to be repeated many times.

There are few jobs in the garden that are not physically challenging, from pruning trees, to mowing the lawn or even pulling out a few weeds. A few moments of thought and planning may save hours of pain and misery. After all, what good is a nice garden if you are not able to go out and enjoy it? The weeds and grass will probably grow much quicker than the time taken to recover from your strained back!

Tips

- Use a narrow spade or fork with a light handle so that there is less weight to each turn of the soil.
- Stop frequently and walk away to do something else in order to allow the muscles to relax.

- If a large area needs to be tackled, divide the area up into realistic pieces and dig one portion each day. It may take longer, but it will pay in the long run.
- Keep your lower back covered with clothing. It will help prevent cold air allowing the back muscles to cool and so become tight.
- Don't bend from the waist to pull up weeds – sit, crouch or kneel in such a way so that your lower back does not have to support your entire upper body weight in a stooping position.
- Use a wheelbarrow to transport heavy pots or plants rather than attempt to carry them.
- Create a raised bed for seedlings or position seed trays on a table or staging to avoid bending down.

Golf

Most sports involve fresh air, exercise and competition. What could be better? Golf is enjoyed by thousands of people across the world, but it is also the cause of countless lower-back injuries. Both the unnatural movement of the golf swing and the repetitive bending and lifting of a heavy golf bag can place excessive stress on the lower back. Younger players can be particularly at risk, since they tend to strike the ball with maximum exertion. Amateur players, particularly, are prone to injury as the action of the golf swing is a violent twisting action. As much as eight times your body weight is forced through the spine. The combination of an imperfect technique, repetitive striking of the ball, and lack of muscular fitness can very often result in serious back pain. It is the spinal joints of the lower back, typically L5-S1 (just below the waist), which suffer injury as this is the joint which mostly allows us to rotate. The thoracic back muscles higher up the torso are also prone to strain.

Players whose sedentary lifestyle may only allow a weekly game and who have not received the benefit of professional training can generate considerable muscle imbalances. This can eventually lead to degenerative disc disease.

Tips

- Always carry out warm-up exercises of stretching, together with smooth and effortless practice swings to stimulate the flexibility of the muscles.

- If you are carrying your clubs, use a bag with two shoulder straps so that the load is evenly distributed across both your shoulders.
- Push rather than pull a wheeled golf trolley to avoid twisting as you walk.

Handbags

The common belief that a woman's handbag holds 'everything but the kitchen sink' may be a gross exaggeration, but nevertheless, they can be very heavy accessories at times. The convenience of a shoulder strap enables the bag to be carried in such a way as to allow both hands to be free to carry other items or perhaps to hold a child's hand. Weight persistently carried in this way, balanced and suspended from one shoulder, not only causes tension in both the shoulder and neck muscles, but can also distort the posture by making one shoulder higher than the other. This imbalance then puts strain on the back muscles, and the result is pain.

Tips

- Try to limit the contents of your handbag to reduce its weight.
- Alternate your bag from one shoulder to the other often, rather than always using the same side, or even tuck the bag under one arm.
- A better alternative, if possible, is to use a back pack, where the weight is supported equally on both shoulders and centrally against your upper back, which is also close to your centre of gravity.

Ironing

Ironing boards which cannot be raised to a comfortable height are also a cause of severe back strain. Not only do you have to lean forward, but the weight of the water-filled iron in one hand whilst manipulating clothes or sheets with the other, helps to place even more stress on the back muscles.

Tips

- When purchasing an ironing board, ensure that it at least extends to between hip and waist height so that your back can be maintained straight throughout the task.

- Consider the weight of the iron you purchase and bear in mind that it will be even heavier when it is full of water. Most manufacturers state the weight of the product on the box.

Pushchairs

Choosing the right pushchair for a new family arrival is both exciting and expensive. The choice is vast and decisions are likely to be made on preference of colour, number of wheels, carrying capacity, and forward or backward facing. But is the model you choose likely to give you back ache, especially when you push it for some distance with a load on board?

Tips

- Consider the height of the handles. If they are much lower than the level of your elbows, it may encourage a stooping posture as you wheel it along.
- Remember too, that as most pushchairs incorporate carrying trays for shopping and as the newborn quickly grows into a sturdy toddler, the weight to be pushed will be greatly increased.

Shoes

Shoe fashions change all the time and it is to our credit and benefit that nowadays softer, flat shoes are more commonly acceptable for women. However, the wearing of high-heeled shoes has always been a sensitive issue, especially for fashion-conscious women. The increased height and undoubted elegance that high-heels present have, over the years, offered a smart appearance in the office workplace and undeniable glamour at social occasions. However, there is a high price to pay for this stylish approach to footwear on a daily basis.

Any heel over 5 centimetres (2 inches) pitches the body forwards so that all the body's weight is placed on the balls of the feet. This means that the toes are unable to propel the body forwards, which is their intended role when walking.

This abnormal stance places unreasonable strain on the lower back, neck and shoulders as well as shortening the calf muscles and damaging the feet.

Tips

- Keep a pair of flat shoes in the car for driving and walking.
- Exercise your back, calves and ankles regularly so that the muscles and tendons can cope with the altered alignment and weight distribution of your body.
- It is advisable to wear high-heeled shoes only for those occasions that really require them.

Shopping

Shopping is so much easier these days for those who have the advantage of driving to large supermarkets where trolleys, convenient parking and assistants are available to help load your bags into your car. On returning home, however, unloading those heavy bags is yet another task that can put your back at risk.

Tips

- Use more bags (re-usable if possible) rather than fewer, so that there is less weight in each.
- Don't twist your body when lifting the bags from the boot. Lift and then turn.
- Although it may take a few minutes longer to unload the car, carry only easily manageable loads at a time.

Sitting at a computer or desk

Sitting for a prolonged period of time, whether it is working at a computer, or doing homework at a desk, or some similar occupation requiring concentration, heightens the risk of developing back pain. It may only be when the task is completed and you attempt to move from your chair that you fully realise the stiffness and rigidity in your back muscles, especially if, during the course of your work, you have been leaning forwards without support to your lower back.

Tips

- A quick exercise to prevent or relieve tension in the neck, shoulders and lower back is easier than you think and does not involve an energetic gymnastic display to interrupt your work!
- Take a moment to sit up as tall as you can, lifting your ribs and tipping your chin slightly downwards so that your neck is straight. Keep looking forwards. Clasp your hands behind your back and pull your shoulders back. This will regain your posture and stretch the muscles away from the slumped and round-shouldered pose that your concentration has allowed you to settle into. Hold this position for a few moments whilst taking slow, deep breaths.
- The improved oxygenation to the muscles will not only refresh your position, but may also improve your function level too.
- Repeat this every 15 minutes or so.

Sneezing

You may wonder why sneezing is included when it is hardly a household chore! It is, however, a very common cause of back pain and unfortunately, not one that we can always avoid.

As well as a head cold, all sorts of things make us sneeze, such as dust, cleaning agents, pet hairs, flour, bright lights, pollen, and sometimes perfume. It is an automatic response to a variety of stimulants, resulting in an almost involuntary projection of released air from the nose. Some say the speed of the release is close to 35-40 miles per hour and others, as much as 100 miles per hour!

Due to its propensity to spread infectious air-borne droplets to a distance of several feet, our instinct is to quickly cover our face and turn away. The spontaneous reaction of twisting to the side, combined with the tremendous force used by the chest muscles to carry out the sneeze, can wrench the back muscles in a split second.

Tips

- Turn the whole of your body so that your back remains straight.
- If possible, turn your whole body or step back and look directly down to the floor in order to reduce the risk of spreading airborne germs.

Vacuum cleaning

For a start, vacuum cleaning is fraught with danger. Upright cleaners certainly reduce the need to twist as the machine can be manoeuvred around the floor by pushing, but there always comes a time when a pipe and nozzle are required to negotiate awkward spaces beneath or behind furniture. This activity can sometimes necessitate stooping and stretching, rather like a caver about to crawl into a tiny cavern. Also, how many times is a chair or similar object moved with one hand whilst wielding the vacuum cleaner with the other?

For those of us who prefer to use a cylinder-type vacuum cleaner, the twisting and need to lean forwards with the brush are even greater.

Tips

- Prepare the room first by exposing areas behind or obscured by furniture so that cleaning these areas is easier. Then replace the items to their original position before doing the central floor area.
- When purchasing a vacuum cleaner, pay particular attention to its weight. There is a tremendous difference according to the type and style available and they can range in weight from about 4 kilograms to over 10 kilograms. This is particularly relevant with the cylinder-type cleaners, which need to be pulled along the floor or carried up stairs.

Work surfaces

Prolonged periods of time spent standing before the kitchen sink or ironing board can be responsible for placing persistent wear on our back muscles. It is easy to dismiss many everyday tasks as insignificant – until the back pain strikes.

It is not the standing, but the forward lean that causes the problem. The usual height of a sink unit can be too low for those slightly above average height. The standard unit itself, with drawer or cupboard doors, does not allow for work to be carried out with one foot placed before the other in a 'walking stance,' which helps us to maintain our centre of gravity (see chapter 9). This means that the weight of our upper body is tipped forwards and the back muscles have to take the strain of maintaining our balance.

Tips

- One solution is to place a plastic washing-up bowl in the sink on top of another up-turned plastic container. Washing up, peeling vegetables, etc, can then be carried out without stooping.
- This is a cheaper solution than altering the kitchen units or digging a hole in the floor to stand in!

Chapter 6

When acute pain becomes chronic

It is widely recognised that acute pain is termed chronic when it has been in existence for three–six months. In the case of back pain, not only does this affect as many as 19% of European adults, but it is also emerging as an increasing problem for children and adolescents, estimated to be even as high as 25% (Breivika H et al 2006). Youngsters aged between 10 and 15 years who participate in sport are particularly at risk of back pain due mostly to muscle strain. Add to this an ever-growing aging population, increasingly sedentary lifestyles, and growing levels of obesity and it is easy to understand how prevalent this problem has become.

The effects of chronic back pain have a tremendous impact on the economy. This is not just a problem in the UK and Europe. For Australia and United States, for example, the costs also run into billions of dollars.

Long-term incapacity, for which many people require disability benefits, is most commonly the result of chronic musculoskeletal disorders, in particular that of non-specific lower back pain. Although the exact cost of chronic pain is unknown, the cost of back pain to the exchequer is estimated to be in excess of £5 billion per annum in the UK (Maniadakis N, Gray A 2000). Its prevention is in everybody's interests. Regardless of the cost to healthcare systems across the world, there is also a very high price to be paid by sufferers and their families in terms of physical, psychological and social wellbeing. Chronic back pain can completely dominate the sufferer's life until there is hardly a minute of the day when pain is not the controlling agent.

Individual experience of pain

Pain is always individual to the sufferer. For those afflicted by back pain, to be told that it may be partly psychological can be very distressing. A patient may also feel that the suffering he/she is experiencing is not being taken seriously enough or even that the person making such a suggestion is opting out of dealing with the problem. However, it has been shown (Loeser J & Melzack R 1999) that the brain recognises both mental and physical pain in much the same way. This means that the body's interpretation of psychological pain can sometimes be confused with that of the back pain, especially if there has been distressing trauma which has resulted in other, more intangible or personal losses. For example, if physical pain is combined with grief or emotional distress, such as the experience of a bad car accident, the physical injury may recover long before the psychological damage is healed. The brain, however, may still perceive pain as though the physical injury still existed.

We all experience pain in different ways. Our pain threshold is determined by a number of genetic and environmental factors. Our gender, culture, social background, upbringing and even our expectations relating to pain, mean that our coping mechanisms are extremely varied. Studies, such as Harding et al 2010, also show that psychosocial issues play a significant part in the transition from acute to chronic pain; these include depression, anxiety and even our attitudes to pain. In the home, financial stress, family relationships, poor housing and bad nutrition can all contribute to back pain becoming a chronic condition.

What's going on? – The importance of getting a diagnosis

There are very many types and causes of back pain and, in general, appropriate treatment and rehabilitation can both restore good mobility and reduce discomfort.

The most common type of back pain is termed 'simple', or 'mechanical', low back pain, which may occasionally radiate to the thighs and buttocks. Because symptoms tend to vary depending upon the type of movement or activity responsible for the pain, it is this variability of symptoms which classifies it as 'mechanical'.

For some, a persistent, aching back can be a problem that comes with increasing age. If there appears to be no identifiable cause or injury, a proper consultation should always be sought from a doctor. This is because it is essential to eliminate the possibility of other, more serious conditions, such as osteoporosis (bone thinning), spinal rigidity caused by the joints of the back losing their mobility and causing a stooping posture, or even cancer. In fact, any back pain which appears to be unrelated to a known back strain or lifestyle cause, should always be examined by a doctor before embarking on a programme of exercise. It is reassuring to know, however, that serious spinal pathology affects only 1% or less of all sufferers.

MRI (magnetic resonance imaging) is often used for diagnosis. However, most back pain is non-specific (85%), which means that it is uncertain where the pain is originating. Although scans may show physical changes due to trauma or the ageing process, it is not necessarily helpful in identifying an actual source of pain. For this reason an MRI scan is generally only used in cases where a surgical operation is being considered or where more sinister causes than the usual back strain or sprain are suspected, owing to other clinical signs.

Violent trauma, which causes serious spinal injuries involving damage to the spinal bones, nerves or blood vessels that supply the spinal cord, is beyond the scope of this book. Such injuries are likely to be the result of road accidents, serious sporting injuries, domestic accidents or perhaps criminal assault. It is, however, important to be aware of a potential serious injury if back pain is the result of a more minor accident or fall. Even moderate damage to the spine, if it produces symptoms of widespread weakness, numbness or bladder dysfunction, should receive professional medical help.

In the majority of cases, the onset of back pain can be traced back to a known movement or strain, perhaps involving lifting a heavy object or wrenching the supporting back muscles. Sometimes, however, in cases of soft tissue injury, the original cause of back strain may be seen to be too trivial to be significant, or even difficult to identify. Even the exact site of the pain may seem difficult to pinpoint; the pain may appear to move from one area to another and be inconsistent in intensity. For some sufferers, as already stated, no specific cause for the pain can be found at all. Back pain that is not resolved should be referred by your general practitioner to an orthopaedic surgeon or pain clinic based in a hospital. . An MRI scan may then be used to identify the problem or to eliminate structural or degenerative causes.

Another possible cause of chronic pain can be the build-up of scar tissue resulting from an earlier injury or previous surgical operation involving the spine. Again, professional medical help will be required to help with this, as reha-bilitative exercises alone may not resolve the problem. This type of problem will also be identified by a spinal surgeon or pain specialist, whereupon appropriate action will be planned. In some cases a small area of scar tissue may be required to be surgically removed to relieve the pressure causing the pain.

Keep moving! – The importance of mobility

Following any minor strain from which back pain results, and during the early acute stage, it is important that a positive programme of movement and exercise is followed. To help you, relevant stretching and strengthening exercises are ex-plained in chapters 11 and 12. It is generally when the acute phase has passed unchecked and the sufferer has become accustomed to making allowances for his/her inability to carry out normal everyday activities that the pain easily slips into a long-standing or chronic problem.

Sufferers who are anxious about their pain will generally resist the increased discomfort of movement because they fear it will exacerbate their problem. By believing that either prolonged complete rest or medication alone will make them better, the likelihood of developing chronic symptoms and long-term disability are greatly increased.

It is human nature to take whatever action we can find to avoid pain. The natural desire to keep perfectly still to avoid aggravating the muscle spasm often means that a distorted alignment is maintained longer than necessary. Sitting crooked on a chair, leaning or limping as we try to walk, can, if it helps at the time, easily become a bad habit. Our normal gait is altered, so that when the pain of the original injury has eventually disappeared, we are still walking like a cartoon character!

The problem with this is that as our alignment becomes more permanently adjusted, strain begins to develop on the limbs and joints that now have to take the extra pressure. Indeed, some patients having presented themselves to the doctor with pain in their knees or hips are sometimes surprised to learn that the initial problem actually lies with their back and the imbalance of weight carried by the spine. If complete restoration of normal mobility is inhibited by the misalignment of the spine, it is likely that the pain will become chronic and the prospect of regaining a full and active life severely affected.

Particular types of chronic back pain

Nerve root pain and lumbar nerve pain are terms often mentioned by doctors in relation to back problems and frequently cause confusion for the lay person.

Nerve root pain

This is when the nerves become pinched or trapped within the spinal column or as they exit from the spine. In addition to pain, the symptoms are tingling, numbness and weakness. The site of the trapped nerve dictates where the symptoms are felt. A nerve trapped in the neck, for example, will give symptoms in the shoulder and arm and those in the lower back will cause pain in the buttock and leg. The pain may be accompanied by feelings of pins and needles, numbness or burning.

Lumbar nerve pain

Lumbar nerve pain is more commonly known as 'sciatica'. One of the common causes of sciatica is a prolapsed or 'slipped' disc, with the resultant pain coming from the nerve trapped by the pressure of the displacement. Whereas common back pain is normally felt between the lower ribs and the buttocks, sciatic pain generally runs in a line from the buttocks, down the centre of the back of the leg, to below the knee. The pain is felt in the lower back, buttock, and/or various parts of the leg and foot. In addition to pain, which is sometimes severe, there may be numbness, muscular weakness, pins and needles or tingling and difficulty in moving or controlling the leg. Sometimes both back and sciatic pain are present at the same time, but the leg pain can be far worse, making it difficult to find any resting position that offers relief.

As well as this common cause, deep inside the buttock is a muscle called the 'piriformis muscle'. It lies right over the sciatic nerve where it exits the spine. Tension in this muscle can also put pressure on the sciatic nerve, with the result that a sharp, stabbing pain radiates the entire length of the nerve down the back of the leg. If the muscle is weak it can make the sciatica worse and prolonged. Exercises to strengthen the abdominal and lower back muscles will help aid recovery, but an accurate diagnosis should first be sought from a doctor or physiotherapist to ensure that the exercises undertaken are appropriate and correctly performed.

Strangely enough, sciatica is more common in 30–40 year olds than in the elderly. This is because as we age, the intervertebral discs become less spongy and are therefore less likely to be forced out of alignment. Unfortunately, there is no 'quick fix' for sciatica, but, having said that, in 90% of patients, sciatic pain due to a prolapsed disc resolves within a reasonable period of time. Analgesic and anti-inflammatory medication, together with gentle stretching exercises, will usually allow complete recovery, although this can sometimes take several weeks. The application of a cold gel pack, or towel soaked in cold water, for up to 10 minutes at a time, may help reduce the pain and inflammation. Avoid sitting for long periods of time, or soaking in a hot bath, since this may exacerbate the sciatic pain by increasing the swelling.

Accurate diagnosis by a doctor, which involves the assessment of power, reflex and sensory tests, will help to identify which nerve is causing the pain, and from this, appropriate treatment can be recommended. This includes medications, interventional injections, surgery or alternative treatments as noted in chapters 13 and 14.. Throughout the treatment, maintaining an active lifestyle, a sensible diet and adequate restful sleep should aid a complete recovery. However, if there is no change after about a month, further professional help may be required.

Key points

- Acute pain is classified as 'chronic' after three–six months.

- Pain is specific to the individual and will generally include a psychological as well as a physical component.

- Proper diagnosis by a health professional is essential before embarking on any sort of treatment, especially where there is no clear cause or identifiable initial trauma.

- Coping strategies in the early stages of acute back pain can contribute to the problem becoming chronic; it is important to keep mobile and be aware how you are compensating for the initial problem.

- Nerve root pain is when the nerve is pinched or trapped either within the spinal column or where it exits the spine.

- Lumbar nerve pain, or 'sciatica', is a distinct type of back pain, generally caused by a prolapsed, or 'slipped', disc; it requires a specific approach to diagnosis and treatment.

References

Breivik H, Collett B, Ventafridda V, Cohen R, Gallacher D. Survey of Chronic Pain in Europe; prevalence, impact on daily life and treatment. *European Journal of Pain* 2006; **10**: 287-333.

Harding G, Campbell J, Parsons S, Rahman A, Underwood M. et al. British pain clinic practitioners' recognition and use of the bio-psychosocial pain management model for patients when physical interventions are ineffective or inappropriate: results of a qualitative study. *BMC Musculoskeletal Disorders* 2010; **11**:51.

Loeser J, Melzack R. Pain: An Overview. *The Lancet* 1999; **353**: 1607–1609.

Maniadakis N, Gray A. The economic burden of back pain in the UK. *Pain* 2000; 84: 95–103.

Wall P, Melzack R. Pain mechanisms: a new theory. *Science* 1965; 150: 971-979.

Chapter 7

When back pain causes depression

As if coping with back pain were not enough, another more insidious problem affects millions of sufferers. Depression may seem to be an unlikely bed-fellow to accompany a painful back but their close association is well documented. A high percentage, averaging 62% (Sinel, Deardorff & Goldstein 1996) of those affected by chronic or long-term back problems also suffer from some type of depressive symptoms. This combination can create havoc with people's lives.

Fortunately, for the vast majority of back pain sufferers, the painful episode is acute and short lived, lasting only for a few days, or a week or two at most. During this time, daily routine is interrupted but following a period of rest, pain-killers and rehabilitative exercise, individuals are usually able to resume their normal activities and put the whole painful experience behind them.

For many others, however, it is not so simple. Back pain can be a difficult condition to treat and, although doctors may do their best and offer every possible medical treatment available to them, in some cases the pain may be stubbornly resistant to all types of therapy.

We all understand that pain is a symptom that something is wrong. We can be forgiven, therefore, for assuming that if conventional treatments have failed to resolve the pain, there must be a more serious cause, but this is not necessarily the case. Conversely, disc herniation (see Figure 2.2, page 9) has occasionally been discovered in individuals with no experience of back pain at all.

X-rays, radiographs, magnetic resonance imaging (MRI scans) and computerised axial tomography studies (CAT scans) are able to identify or eliminate any anatomical changes or abnormalities that might necessitate invasive surgery or other treatment, but they cannot always reveal the cause of the pain. Over a period of years, some patients try a proliferation of both medical and complementary treatments in the hope of banishing the pain and yet it persists, leading to feelings of despair and hopelessness.

The downward spiral

To understand this situation, it is necessary to examine the way in which back pain can affect not just the individual, but also other family members and close friends.

Frustration, perhaps, is the first emotion when normal activities, such as dressing or picking up an object from the floor, can cause such pain as to make even the simplest of activities almost impossible. Frustration, sometimes anger, can eventually give way to an acceptance that the only relief is immobility.

Some people may find lying down reasonably comfortable, but for many, sleep is almost impossible as no position can give relief for very long. The resulting fatigue can then lead to irritability the following day. Not only does this have a further detrimental effect on the sufferer, but it can adversely affect the partner, if his/her sleep has also been disturbed.

The enduring incapacity caused by back pain can be extremely stressful, further compounded by the need for other family members to carry out the tasks normally managed by the sufferer. Movement becomes slow and careful, with the sufferer not wanting to antagonise the back muscles; there is then little incentive to leave the home. Avoiding further discomfort becomes a priority. Social activities and meeting with friends eventually cease, leading to loneliness and loss of independence.

For the sufferer, this feels like a self-perpetuating downward physical and emotional spiral. Without the ability to work, care for the children or participate in leisure pursuits previously enjoyed, this can change a formerly positive and lively individual by forcing him/her into reclusive isolation.

Stress begins to put pressure on the whole household. This, in turn, causes the back pain to increase and many turn to comfort-eating as a means of acquiring that 'feel good' effect that can't now be got from previously enjoyed activities. Inevitably, without the ability to exercise, weight increases, the pain remains unrelenting, and depression sets in. Long-term sick leave, with no certainty of returning to work, can eventually result in loss of employment and the financial situation of the household can be dramatically affected. Family relationships suffer and sexual activity is probably the last thing on the sufferer's mind, which can again cause more stress.

This is a very bleak picture, but it is an important point to make. It is easy to see why positive action is best taken at the very onset of back pain. When its presence becomes the dominating factor, it can so easily trap a sufferer in a more permanent cycle of pain.

Some researchers claim that there is a 'chicken and egg' situation here. Individuals with back pain suffer depression because of a physical pain, whilst others suffer back pain as a result of depression. Either way, it would appear to be the loss of control that overwhelms the sufferer, leading him/her into this downward spiral. For this reason, expert professional help is required and the help and encouragement of those close to the sufferer can be of enormous benefit. Recovery is greatly improved by a positive attitude towards rehabilitative exercise and mobility, which are essential as soon as the problem is recognised.

Key points

- 62% of patients with chronic back pain also develop depressive symptoms.

- Pain is not necessarily proportionate to the underlying injury and severe back pain may have no clear physical cause or cure.

- With chronic back pain comes a downward spiral from frustration, to anger, to exhaustion, to depression.

- Family members will also be affected.

- Back pain and depression are closely linked, with loss of control being a key factor.

- Positive action at the onset of back pain is essential for avoiding the downward spiral.

Reference

Sinel MS, Deardorff WW, Goldstein TB. *Win the Battle Against Back Pain – an integrated approach.* USA: Dell, 1996.

Chapter 8

Assessing the risk

Outside the home everything we do these days seems to require a 'risk assessment'. We hear all the time how businesses and employees alike are instructed to carry out these reviews, for which written documentation often has to be completed. In the workplace this might be an obligatory requirement under Health and Safety legislation, but no one is suggesting that such a procedure should ever be carried out formally in the home. However, the same principles apply to any physical task, wherever we are.

You may not realise it, but the fact is we generally carry out risk assessments several times a day, usually subconsciously and often in the blink of an eye. This may sound improbable, but it is nothing more than instinctive self-preservation.

Take crossing the road, for instance. There are four important factors that we consider to ensure that we reach the other side safely, and these are just the same factors that will determine our safety when carrying out any other physical activity.

These four factors are the **'task'** itself, or our intention; our **'individual capability'**; the **'load'**, or most important component of the job from a risk point of view; and the **'environment'** in which we intend to carry it out.

Just crossing the road will automatically bring all four of these factors into play:

1. The '**task**' we have set ourselves is to get across to the other side safely.
2. Our **individual capability** takes into account our personal fitness and ability to get across – that is, can we walk quickly? Do we have the encumbrance of a push chair or shopping with us? Do we need to walk slowly with a stick? The speed we are capable of dictates our time and ability to get across the road.

3. The **load**, or major risk factor, can be seen as the volume of traffic, its speed and whether there are many large vehicles at the time.

4. The **environment** can be seen as whether the road surface is wet or slippery with ice, or whether the light is poor or visibility restricted by either a nearby corner in the road or parked vehicles.

Omit any one of these four elements when assessing the task of crossing the road and we're likely to get run over!

The fact that we can safely manage such a potentially dangerous manoeuvre thousands of times, in all sorts of places, and in many different circumstances, shows that we are actually pretty good at making risk assessments. Unfortunately, we all too often fail to apply such good practice to our everyday, more mundane household chores and as a consequence, suffer pain and injury for our apathy.

Applying the four components of risk assessment to our other everyday activities should be as automatic and instinctive as when we cross the road. We just have to learn to ask ourselves a few questions about the task we intend to carry out. Although it is never possible completely to avoid unforeseen accidents, by using and remembering this easy mnemonic, TILE (task, individual capability, load, and environment), the risk of harming our backs will be vastly reduced.

In addition, when considering any action, we should not just look at the individual task but acknowledge other influential factors, such as how often the task needs to be performed or how long the required exertion will take. Laying slabs for a patio, for example, will require the same actions to be carried out many times and it is the repetitive nature of such a job that is likely to cause back strain.

Risk assessment in practice

Outlined below are considerations and questions that may help you avoid some of the dangers you encounter every day. You may have to force yourself to take these into account consciously at first, but practice will mean they become second nature to you, just like crossing the road.

The task itself

Q: Am I likely to stoop? For example, when lifting a heavy washing basket from the floor.

Q: Will it make me twist? For example, when sweeping snow to the side of the path.

Q: Have I got to carry a heavy load far? For example, purchases from shops to the car park.

Q: Will I be reaching upwards repetitively? For example, painting and decorating.

Q: Will I be pushing or pulling an excessive load? For example, a family member in a wheelchair.

Q: Will this task require frequent or prolonged physical effort? For example, vacuuming, polishing furniture, gardening.

Breaking the task down into its component parts, or reducing the amount of time spent at any one stage, can in some cases be helpful. Does all the housework need to be done in one day? Can a variety of diverse jobs in the garden, each requiring different activities, be done instead of doing all the digging in one session? Smaller, more realistic targets are easier to achieve and help prevent the strain of repetitive actions.

Your individual capability

Our physical ability to manage many everyday activities depends mostly on factors such as our age and general health. Instinctively we recognise whether certain tasks are easily manageable or whether they may require the assistance of another person.

Due to the different muscle densities of males and females, the maximum safe weight that can be carried by women is only two thirds of that which can be managed by men. This figure is further reduced when muscle mass and bone strength decline in our later years – that is, women lose proportionately more with age than do men.

The maximum safe weight that we should attempt to lift will also depend upon whether we are able to take hold of the load at waist height. If the object to be carried is already positioned at shoulder height or even higher, or perhaps placed down on the floor, again the maximum load is considerably reduced (see Figure 8.1).

A further consideration is whether we are able to hold the weight close against our body or whether this is inappropriate due to the nature of the load. A weight

Table 8.1 National guidance for the maximum weight an 'average' person can lift, showing how this is reduced by height and distance from the lifter. (This assumes the maximum for men is 25 kg and for women 15 kg, but this will vary according to the individual's fitness.)

	Women		Men	
	Close to body	Away from body	Close to body	Away from body
Shoulder height	7 kg	3 kg	10 kg	5 kg
Elbow height	13 kg	7 kg	20 kg	10 kg
Knuckle height with arms straight down	15 kg	10 kg	25 kg	15 kg
Mid lower leg height	13 kg	7 kg	20 kg	10 kg
Ground	7 kg	3 kg	10 kg	5 kg

that we may feel comfortable to lift and which can comfortably be held against the body to be carried for a short distance, will not strain our backs as much as an awkwardly shaped or bulky item that is difficult to hold but of similar weight.

Our general fitness and, in particular, any previous history of back injury, will inevitably affect our ability to tackle the most strenuous of tasks. Extra care must be taken if there has been a recent episode of back pain or if symptoms of strain are already present. Sometimes, the most obvious and sensible solution - of waiting for someone else to give assistance – is banished in our impatience to get the job done, but it can prove to be a costly error of judgement.

For some tasks, such as moving furniture, digging up and moving a small tree, or maybe retrieving items from a loft space, it is always safer with a second person's help. But don't forget that it is important to be just as concerned for his/her safety, also taking into consideration his/her general health, age and height.

It is sometimes difficult to co-ordinate a good lift with a second person whose height is vastly different from your own, since the balance of weight carried will be unequal. Even if only a short distance is to be covered, the load may well be unsafe. Always discuss the task to be achieved, ensuring that the easiest method possible is used. It may well be that a trolley or wheelbarrow can be used to make the task safer, or you can agree a point at which the load will be rested and you will both be able to take a few moments' respite.

When moving a heavy object, such as a piece of furniture, it is imperative that you work in unison. Before starting the lift, agree the commands that will be used and decide who will give them. Do not be tempted to use, 'One, two, three'. The problem with this command is that one person will lift the object on the word 'three' while the other may assume the unspoken word 'four', and the lift itself will be uneven and potentially dangerous. In this instance, the first person will attempt to lift the object on his/her own a moment before the second person. It is likely that the first person will drop the item because it is too heavy just as the second person takes the weight. In this way, both parties are likely to give themselves a strained back.

The ideal command, agreed in advance, is that of **'ready, brace, move'**. The word 'ready' denotes the moment to clasp the object firmly, with both knees bent, back straight and looking forwards in preparation for the lift. The use of the second word, 'brace', signals the time to engage the abdominal muscles by pulling them in towards the spine. The last command, 'move', leaves no doubt that this is the moment to take the strain and co-ordinate the joint manoeuvre.

Suitable loose (but not flowing) clothing and flat shoes are always helpful to ensure both freedom of movement and that the weight of your body is well balanced in relation to the ground.

The load
The load, or weight, can be either a person or an object.

When the load is an object
If it is an inanimate object that you wish to move, again there are several questions you may wish to consider:

Q: Is the load marked with its weight and centre of gravity? For example, heavy delivery items will usually have the weight of the box printed on them.

Q: Is it bulky or unwieldy? For example, the object may not be heavy, but can you get a good grip of it and see over the top to where you are going?

Q: Is it fragile? For example, is it a box of crockery, or a television?

Q: Is it intrinsically harmful? For example, is it a pan of hot jam, or a pane of glass?

When the load is another person

Carrying a small child can be difficult and, for most mothers, is an activity undertaken many times every day. Assisting an elderly relative in the home can also be extremely taxing and the resultant repetitive actions are a common cause of back strain. Again, some fundamental questions need consideration:

Q: What is the weight and size of the child? Small children are constantly growing and getting heavier. The temptation to sit a toddler across one hip so that you have a free hand for picking up a bag or opening a door with the other is one of the most common causes of back strain in young mothers.

Q: How able is the youngster to cooperate? Is he/she likely to throw his/her weight away from your body and centre of gravity, so that your back has to take the unexpected strain to prevent you both from falling?

Q: How mobile is your elderly relative? For example, can he/she weight-bear and understand instructions which will assist you when helping him/her out of a chair or bed?

Q: How able is the elderly relative to cooperate? For example, does pain or spasm restrict his/her movement, which may cause sudden and unpredictable resistance to the planned move?

Above all, be very aware of your own limitations. It is of no help to those you are attempting to help if you sustain an injury that may take several weeks to recover from. If you are nursing a relative at home, never be afraid to seek advice or ask for help if you need it. Remember, a move that is badly managed because the task is too great for you, may also result in pain, discomfort, or even injury, for the person you are caring for.

The environment

It may sound unnecessarily fussy to worry about where you are or your immediate surroundings when managing everyday tasks in the home, but it can make a big difference in relation to your back care.

Q: Are you in a restricted space? For example, making a bed or moving an object in order to clean behind it. Although it is not possible to change the shape or size of your rooms, excessive clutter (and we all have some) could perhaps be rearranged so that it is possible to pull a bed away from the wall, or even position it so that you have access on both sides. This is particularly important when caring for a disabled or elderly relative.

Q: Can casters be fitted to the feet of appliances to make them easier to slide in and out? Preparation of the most challenging tasks is half the battle.

Q: Is it too hot or cold? This may sound silly, but being encumbered by too much thick clothing can restrict movement. On the other hand, loose flowing summer garments can present a hazard if they become inadvertently caught or trapped so that your action is jarred as a result.

Q: Is the floor or ground surface uneven and free of objects? For example, are there rugs, door thresholds or toys likely to cause you to trip? Water, too, may make the surface slippery.

Q: Is there sufficient light? For example, can you see properly to identify whether there are any deviations in the floor level, or whether a flex is lying across your line of travel?

Q: Is there any equipment available which might make your job easier? This could be a sack, trolley or wheel-barrow, for example. Hoists, handrails, bath seats or specially designed showers and many other pieces of equipment are available for those looking after a disabled or elderly relative at home.

Positive conclusion

Learning to assess the risk to your safety takes only a moment. By pausing just long enough to identify potential dangers and, if necessary, changing the way each task is physically tackled, can make all the difference. You may be surprised how quickly you not only recognise poor technique in some of your regular actions but how safer methods soon become habitual, so that you no longer even consciously think about it. In the same way that you would not dream of crossing a busy road without taking account of approaching traffic, even crouching down rather than stooping to pick up a piece of paper from the floor will become second nature to you.

Key points

- We assess risk many times a day without realising it but often fail to do so for tasks that we think of as relatively undemanding.

- The key factors when assessing risk are the **task**, our **individual capability**, the **load**, and the **environment** – remember, 'TILE'.

- For our backs we must also factor in the duration and repetitiveness of the task.

- If lifting with someone else, planning an agreed approach and unambiguous command will significantly reduce the risks... .

- ... as will learning to ask ourselves key questions about any lifting task.

- Over time doing so will become second nature and we will hardly notice how carefully we are protecting our backs.

Chapter 9

The principles of moving and handling

What does 'moving and handling' mean? It is basically the physical action we need to take in order to lift or move an object or person from one place to another, or to carry out a practical task. This includes lifting, lowering, pushing, pulling and carrying. The fundamental principles are easy to learn and depend simply on planning ahead and maintaining good posture throughout the movement.

In the workplace the word 'ergonomics' is used to describe the scientific discipline that examines the effectiveness and efficiency of workers' activities. The aim of employers is to increase safety, reduce fatigue and stress, and improve comfort in order to increase job satisfaction. In just the same way, the wellbeing of our backs outside the workplace can be greatly improved by just applying a few simple strategies and techniques. The most effective of these is good posture.

Your posture

Good posture is the most important feature of back care. It is both a natural and an efficient stance for the human frame and has advantages other than just good balance. By keeping your bones and joints in proper alignment, it ensures that your muscles are used correctly. This in turn reduces the stress on the ligaments that connect to the spinal joints. By minimising the wear and tear on joint surfaces caused by careless actions, even the risk of future arthritis can be reduced.

During early childhood and our formative years we have naturally good posture and balance. Most of us, unfortunately, develop bad habits over time. Correct posture means that whether we are standing, sitting or lying down, our bodies are able to maintain good alignment and balance so that our centre of gravity is not compromised. Not only does good posture give us a sense of wellbeing and an elegant appearance, but our more effective use of energy also helps to reduce fatigue.

Standing

Standing for long periods of time often causes back pain. This is due to the muscles that support the body becoming tired and collapsing down, allowing the curvature of the spine to become exaggerated. The head tilts forwards, the shoulders slump, the tummy relaxes and the bottom protrudes in order to compensate for the unbalanced weight.

Another commonly adopted stance that causes back trouble involves standing with your weight predominantly on one foot, whilst lightly resting the other on the ground. As your pelvis is tilted sideways, your torso is also twisted and your distribution of weight is again uneven. Although the stance can be altered, and your weight exchanged onto your other foot, the general balance (or rather, imbalance) of your body is reversed and after a while this can become very tiring.

If your posture has become lazy in this way, you need to re-train it by consciously adopting a good stance at all times until this becomes second nature. This does not mean standing stiffly to attention, but learning how to adjust your position to best effect.

One of the best methods of attaining an ideal standing posture is to imagine a piece of string pulling you up from the top of your head. As you hold your head up, keep your chin in, so that your head is balanced and in line with the centre of your body. With shoulders held back, allow them to relax and drop down. There is a great temptation to hunch your shoulders in an effort to gain height, but it is important to consciously resist that strained and 'rounded' position. With your feet slightly apart, lift up your rib cage and slightly tilt your pelvis forwards. Pull your tummy in towards your spine. This may all sound like the actions of a contortionist, but usually only a minor adjustment to your normal pose is required. This is the most natural and balanced position which the human frame

Figure 9.1 Healthy posture
– this is the most natural and
balanced way to stand.

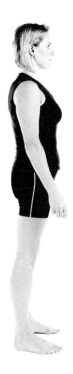

was designed to adopt. Practice and self-awareness will quite quickly make this an instinctive stance, which will reap enormous benefits to your whole physical appearance and attitude (see Figure 9.1).

There are also other benefits to a good and upright posture. The large flat muscle called the 'diaphragm' lies like a slightly domed plate across the centre of your body cavity, just below your ribs. Its job is to contract downwards and, together with the muscles that lie between the ribs, allow them to pivot outwards and upwards thus expanding your chest volume, and draw air (oxygen) into your lungs. A slumped posture and rounded shoulders clearly restrict the efficiency of this process, resulting in a reduced supply of oxygen to the main muscles of your body. This in turn greatly increases the likelihood of fatigue, stiffness and possible muscle spasm.

Digestion is also improved. Poor posture, where your upper body is slumped onto and supported solely by your abdominal organs, instead of by the girdle of muscles designed for the purpose, can make the whole digestive system sluggish and less efficient. The resulting feeling of tiredness removes the incentive to take

Figure 9.2 Healthy posture
– this is the most natural and
balanced way to sit.

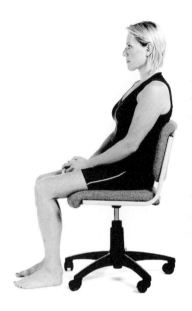

regular exercise and the situation is perpetuated by a sedentary lifestyle and possible weight gain.

Sitting

Sitting also requires good posture. Whether you are working or relaxing, taking the weight off your feet is no reason to collapse into a slumped heap! Ideally, your back should be straight, shoulders back and your buttocks touching the back of the chair. The chair back itself should allow you to maintain the 'S' shape of your spine and support your lumbar region. Your feet should be able to be flat on the floor and the weight of your body evenly distributed over both hips. Your thighs should run parallel to the floor (see Figure 9.2). This may sound difficult to maintain while concentrating on other matters for long periods of time, such as when using the computer or doing homework, but it is important not to relax to the point that you begin to slouch.

If you do so, about every 10 minutes draw yourself up whilst taking in a long deep breath. Exaggerate the lumbar curve and hold it for a few seconds before relaxing slightly. No one position should be held for more than 30 minutes, so stand up and move around in order to mobilise your back muscles.

Try not to sit twisted. Sitting at a desk with the computer screen angled to one side, or watching a television from a poorly positioned chair, will also put unnecessary strain on the muscles on one side. Crossing your legs is also bad for you. Not only does it restrict the circulation to your lower legs, but it again allows a distorted sideways alignment of your spine.

Modern soft sofas sometimes offer little in the way of good lumbar support. Try to sit with your buttocks as far back as possible to the back of the chair and if necessary place a cushion in the small of your back. The temptation to collapse for hours in front of the television can put an enormous amount of strain on your lower back, which will eventually cause discomfort.

It is worth remembering that we are not designed to spend long periods of time either sitting or standing, but it is a fact that these days many of us spend over 90% of our day inactive.

Lifting

Lifting any object effectively and safely also requires good posture. In industry, wherever possible, every effort is made to avoid the need to lift at all by the provision of equipment and devices designed for the purpose. In a busy family home, of course, this is impossible. Generally, the only exception to this is where hoists or sit-in baths can be installed for the disabled or elderly. We therefore need to adopt sensible strategies for the activities we perform in order to prevent injury.

For both men and women, the maximum weight that may be carried should always be held close to the body and at waist or elbow height. For men, this should not exceed 25 kilograms and for women, 15 kilograms. To put this into perspective, a large sack of potatoes is approximately 25 kilograms and the average weight of a three-year-old child is about 15 kilograms. Remember also that where possible these weight limits must be reduced if a load necessitates holding the object above or below waist height or away from the body. For example, the maximum weight suggested that a woman should lift from the floor is only 5 kilograms (see Figure 9.3).

Of course, there are obvious exceptions to this rule. There are very many men who have undertaken strenuous employment, such as farming or building, that has routinely involved heavy lifting throughout their lives. They will claim that they have never experienced pain from back strain. Clearly in these people, muscle strength has been increased over time and their overall fitness has

Figure 9.3 Maximum safe weights to lift – for a woman, 15kg overall but only 5kg if lifting from the floor or holding away from the body. (For a man, 25kg, 10kg and 10kg.)

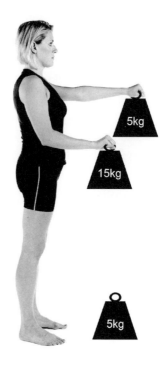

protected them against injury. For the rest of us, the isolated and spontaneous act of reaching to the floor to pick up a piece of paper can occasionally spell disaster!

Before lifting anything, we need to have an awareness of our centre of gravity. If you stand straight with your arms by your sides, the centre of gravity is an imaginary line from the top of your head, down through the middle of your body to the ground beneath your feet. Now, in the same way that a wine glass would topple over without a wide base to support its stem, we too need to increase the size of our base before attempting to lift a weight. To do this, place one foot in front of the other, just as though you were walking and stopped in mid-stride. Your centre of gravity remains unchanged but your stability is greatly improved. Do not be tempted to position your feet apart widthways, since that will make you 'front heavy' when you lift and immediately place a strain on your back muscles (see Figure 9.4).

Next, it is imperative that we make best use of our abdominal muscles. To do this, pull your tummy in as though you want your navel to touch your spine. Engaging these muscles in this way will ensure they support both your back and

Figure 9.4 Preparing to lift a weight – having one foot forward would help to maintain your centre of gravity or balance.

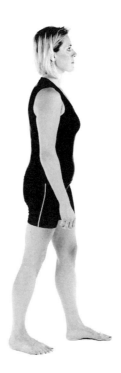

your thigh muscles, so that both power and balance are properly utilised to cope with the anticipated task.

Lift the object as close as you can to your body, making sure that you have a good, firm grip before attempting the lift. Push up with your legs, allowing the strength of your thigh muscles to take the strain. Do not be tempted to look down at the object, but look up slightly so that your neck is not bent. This is particularly important as it will improve your balance and control of the weight. Lastly, do not flex your back as you lift. This happens if you start to straighten your legs before you have taken the weight of the load from the ground.

It is wise to know exactly what you are going to do with your load once you have hold of it. That may sound daft, but once it is in your grasp it may not be easy to open a door or move an object, such as a chair, out of the way in order to make a clear passage way. Balancing or shifting the load to one side in order to free up one hand to undertake a different task may not only make the job more difficult, but more dangerous.

Always lift close to your body, where your strength and stability are greatest.

Keeping your feet apart, one in front of the other, bend your knees and keep your back straight. Pull in your abdominal muscles and take hold of the object with a secure hand grip. Always face the direction of the move, so as not to twist. Look forwards, not down at the object. This will help to maintain the natural curvature of your spine and prevent you from creating a stooping posture.

Taking hold of an object in a jerky or rushed manner will risk you losing your composure. Move smoothly and stay in control. Push up using your thigh muscles as these muscles are much stronger than your back.

It is not always possible to calculate accurately the weight of the load you intend to pick up. Children do not come with a weight label printed on their forehead. But if, as you start to take the force of the weight of an object, you find you need to strain to lift it, gently abandon the move and get help – or wait for it. There are no prizes for being a martyr!

Key points

- Good posture – standing, sitting or lifting – is the most effective way to protect your back.

- Good posture also improves our digestion, energy levels, appearance and sense of wellbeing.

- If you've developed bad posture habits, you will need to consciously re-train yourself until good posture becomes automatic.

- As a general rule, women should not try to lift anything over 15 kilograms, and men, anything over 25 kilograms, and then only if conditions are optimal.

- Balance and power are the key – be aware of your centre of gravity and engage your abdominal and thigh muscles to support your back.

Chapter 10

Movements to avoid

To understand the injuries that may result from certain movements we perform, we need to look again at the structures that are involved. The two most common causes of back pain are muscle 'strain' and muscle 'sprain'. Although different tissues are involved in each case, both conditions display similar symptoms and the treatment is the same for both (see chapter 11).

A **strain** occurs when the muscle itself is over-stretched or even torn. This means that damage occurs to the fibres that make up the muscles, which in turn are made up of chains of muscle cells tightly grouped together.

The muscles are attached to bones by tough fibrous connecting tissue called ligaments. It is when these ligaments are over-stretched or torn that the injury is called a **sprain**.

In order to prevent such stress-related injuries, it is important to recognise that there is a big difference between the amount someone can physically manage to lift and that which is safe to lift. The only prize for attempting to lift too heavy a load is back pain! It may also be disappointing to learn that actions which you have carried out automatically and repetitively for years are just as likely to cause you harm as unaccustomed actions, even when you have previously never suffered as a result. Whilst you may have got away with using somewhat hazardous techniques for as long as you can remember, in the same way that an elastic band will eventually perish and snap, your back muscles and interverte-bral discs may in time protest with a vengeance.

Stooping, twisting and heavy or frequent lifting are perhaps the most obvious movements to avoid, but there are others. Whole-body vibration, for example, as in long-distance driving, is responsible for a great deal of lower back pain. Kneeling whilst leaning forwards and without support is another unsafe action, which is often carried out by gardeners. Postural stress, caused by a high spinal load, occurs when something is held above head height, as in decorating. These are all high risk movements.

Stooping and how to avoid it

Stooping while working

One of the most common actions that put our backs under unnecessary strain is that of working with a constant slight stoop. We are all different shapes and sizes and, just as importantly, different heights. Household equipment and kitchen design, however, are generally made to standard dimensions (unless you are lucky enough to design your own work areas). Consequently, for many taller individuals the preparation of food, say, and washing-up, are always carried out with a slightly stooping posture.

Now before you rush away to dig a trench all around the work areas in your kitchen in order to lower the floor relative to your work surface, or wreck the units by trying to adjust the level of the worktops, there are cheap and easy solutions to make life easier – and safer.

If you wash up or prepare vegetables at the sink, use a plastic washing-up

Figure 10.1 Lifting from the floor – how not to do it.

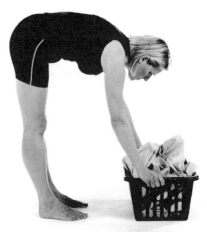

Figure 10.2 Lifting from the floor – how to do it.

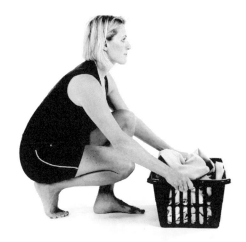

bowl placed on top of another up-turned flat plastic tray (or other suitable item) to raise the level of the water to a height where you no longer need to lean forwards. As with the worktops, a piece of veneered or melamine-covered chipboard placed on the work-surface when you intend to make pastry or chop vegetables, for example, will raise the height by anything from 1–2 centimetres, which may make all the difference to your posture whilst working.

Sudden, quick stooping

We are all guilty of spontaneously stooping to pick something up from the floor without a second thought, but even something as small and light as a piece of paper or a child's toy may result in injury. In this instance it is not so much the size or weight of the object, but the weight of our upper body as it is suddenly propelled forwards. Our centre of gravity is altered away from our normal stance, thus putting all the strain on our back muscles and spine as they endeavour to control our balance, even for just a few moments. Stooping in this way routinely will eventually cause the back muscles to complain and, once again, it's 'Ooh, my back' (see Figure 10.1).

To avoid harm, put one foot in front of the other, bend at the knees to keep your back straight and look forwards. To start with, this may seem a bit over-dramatic and unnecessary, especially if the item you're picking up is very small and light (see Figure 10.2), but learning to do this as a matter of course could save you weeks of pain.

Problem tasks that involve stooping

Emptying the washing machine, pulling the garments from the back of the drum, is also frequently carried out without thought to its potential danger. With one foot in front of the other (so that you don't fall over), crouch down so that the washing machine drum is at eye-level. This not only protects your spine, but also has the added bonus of allowing you to spot that odd sock that loves to adhere to the back of the drum out of sight! This advice will also apply to loading and emptying a dishwasher.

Cleaning the bath is another household task famous for inflicting back pain. Try kneeling on the floor and using your free hand to support your upper body weight as you reach to the far side of the bath. This way your body is adequately braced, especially if you rest your waist on the nearside of the bath at the same time. Twisting or leaning sideways is particularly hazardous and should always be avoided, especially when your back is bent.

Twisting

Whatever you are doing, try not to twist. Face towards the task you are doing, with your shoulders level and in line with your hips. Spread your feet apart to maintain a good balance. If you need to turn, it is better to do so using your feet than to rotate your body whilst carrying a load.

A common hazard is that of suddenly turning your upper body, perhaps when your attention is drawn to something or someone behind you. This may sound silly, but is yet another common cause of muscle strain. Sometimes the inclination to twist is so instinctive that the resultant sideways pull on the muscles is difficult to avoid. By improving the strength and flexibility of the back muscles, using the exercises described later in the book (see chapter 12), this will greatly reduce the risk of harm.

Repetitive actions

Repetitive actions, particularly those involving heavy lifting, are another activity to avoid. Your muscles become tired, your breathing less effective, and an aching back is the first sign of injury. It is sometimes not until the job is finished that the full painful impact of the task is recognised; you will reduce the risk of injury and spot trouble more quickly if you stop for frequent rests.

Reaching up and bending

They say that the kitchen is the most dangerous room in the house. Cookers, electrical white goods, and smooth, shiny or wet floors are probably the obvious hazards one thinks of. But our neat and tidy cupboards are full of awkward, fragile and sometimes heavy objects which are capable of causing us to hurt our backs. An array of cupboards both elevated above the worktop and those from waist height to the floor mean that we store everything either above shoulder height or down at knee height. Reaching up high for several heavy dinner plates, or bending down for a copper-bottomed saucepan, are just the sort of tasks that can cause us strain.

Ideally the best height at which to pick up something heavy is waist level, but this is clearly not always possible. Give consideration to the position and weight of casseroles, saucepans, food tins and crockery. Reorganise, if necessary, by making things as easily accessible as possible. This will both help prevent injury and make your kitchen a more pleasant place in which to work.

Fixed positions

The most subtle cause of back strain is maintaining one fixed position for too long. Sitting watching the television for a lengthy period, particularly in a soft chair that offers insufficient support to your lower back, places great stress on those muscles that are ill equipped to take the constant strain. Although your upper back and shoulders may be resting against the back of the chair, the area around your hips is actually taking most of the weight of your upper body. Slumping in front of a computer, or leaning forwards towards a desk to write, are also invitations to your muscles to become stressed.

You could be forgiven, at this point, for believing that our bodies are not very well designed in the first place, to leave us so vulnerable to back injury. However, it is our lifestyle, and not the structure we are born with, that puts us at so much risk. Washing machines, cars, computers and televisions were not allowed for when we first learnt to walk on two legs!

Key points

- The two most common causes of back pain are muscle strain and muscle sprain

- Movements that are risks for these injuries include:

  - Stooping, either quickly and suddenly, or unsupported for a period while we work;

  - Twisting;

  - Heavy lifting, especially if this is frequent;

  - Repetitive movements and lifting;

  - Reaching up, including holding something heavy above head height;

  - Working at the wrong height so that you have to stoop or reach up repetitively.

- Activities that need to be avoided or undertaken with awareness and care include:

  - Painting/decorating higher than head height;

  - Driving long distance, causing whole-body vibration;

  - Stooping to pull clothes out of the washing machine;

  - Stooping to load or unload a dishwasher;

  - Stooping to clean the bath;

  - Chopping food at a work surface which is too low.

Chapter 11

How to alleviate back pain

Pain is a symptom – a sign that something is wrong. In the case of back pain it is impossible to ignore. It grips like a vice, can cause you to catch your breath and restricts your movement in a way that dramatically inhibits your ability to change position or walk normally. Despite all the positive recommendations to encourage movement and progressive exercise, when back pain strikes, the overwhelming desire is to keep perfectly still to avoid exacerbating the agonising spasm. But we can't stay like a statue for ever.

There are four main components to an effective recovery plan following the onset of a muscle injury or strain:

- Initially, it is good to rest to prevent further deterioration of the tissues for perhaps as long as a day or two.
- Secondly, while resting, apply heat and/or cold to help the damaged area to relax and allow healing to commence. The application of a hot compress will aid the relaxation of the tight muscles, whilst a cold pad helps to reduce inflammation caused by the injury. Alternating this treatment can be very beneficial, but care must be taken to protect the skin from extremes of temperature.
- Next, take appropriate analgesia (pain relief – see below) and then,
- Finally, and most importantly, re-introduce gentle movement and stretching exercises as **soon** as you feel able.

Whatever the cause of the injury, your body has suffered a trauma. As a consequence, the nerve endings in the area affected transmit signals to the brain which you feel as pain. Depending on the severity of the injury, your body will instinctively restrict movement in order to protect itself and prevent further damage. Your own anxiety and fear will add to this and can exacerbate the response by increasing muscle tension. It can even make you believe that you may have suffered permanent harm, especially if the initial pain is severe.

1. Rest

Initially, if the muscles are in spasm, it is sensible to rest until this subsides and a little movement is tolerable . Sitting or lying in a well-supported and comfortable position will allow your muscles to relax. At this time, slow deep breathing will encourage an increased supply of oxygen to penetrate the fibres that have been damaged.

2. Applying hot and/or cold

Heat, perhaps provided by a hot towel, heat pad or hot water bottle, will aid relaxation and increase the blood supply to the affected area. A word of warning – a soak in a hot bath may sound very tempting, but don't forget that you have to both climb in and, more painfully, climb out again, which, if the spasm is bad, may leave you in a very awkward situation! A shower is both a safer and a less stressful option.

Also, a cold compress is recommended to reduce the pain and inflammation of soft tissue injuries. This works by reducing the sensitivity of the nerves, in that the impulses which would have been transmitted from the damaged area are greatly diminished. Ice cubes or a packet of frozen peas, which must be wrapped inside a towel or similar, can be held against the affected area, but for not more than 10 minutes at a time, as increased tension created by the chill can sometimes be counter-productive.

Alternating hot and cold, allowing 10 minutes of each, can be very beneficial. As the blood vessels dilate (get bigger) with the application of heat and contract (get smaller) with the cold compress, damaged cells are more quickly removed from the painful area. This is due to the stimulation of the blood supply to the affected area.

3. Pain-killers

Medication, in the form of pain-killers, is an important part of early treatment. Following back strain, it is helpful to understand the types and strengths of the various analgesics available and the way they work.

Analgesics are divided into two main groups. Firstly, there are the 'simple analgesics', which include paracetamol and the 'non-steroidal anti-inflammatory drugs' – aspirin and ibuprofen. The second group are known as 'opiates'; they are legally controlled, must be prescribed by doctors, and are used only for moderate to severe pain. These include weaker opioids like codeine; intermediate ones like tramadol; and strong varieties like morphine and oxycodone.

The simple analgesics, or 'non-opiates', are less powerful and some are readily available for purchase as 'over-the-counter' medication, without a doctor's prescription. Self-administration of these analgesics is safe provided the manufacturer's guidelines are carefully observed.

The majority of medications take approximately 30 minutes to reach their optimum effect. It is therefore a good idea to take analgesia half an hour prior to introducing some early gentle exercises; the pain will be reduced, allowing much greater movement to be tolerated. The most commonly used are described below.

Paracetamol alone and in combination

Paracetamol is a simple non-opiate analgesic with a low-dependence rating. It is highly regarded as a first choice for mild to moderate pain and is one of the safest when used correctly. It does not tend to irritate the stomach and has very few side effects.

Combination drugs

There are several analgesics that are known as 'combination drugs'. Most of these analgesics contain paracetamol together with another supportive drug, combined to give more effective pain relief. These can usually be identified by the prefix 'co' in the name, as in co-codamol or co-dydramol. The suffix 'amol' at the end of the name is a further indication that part of the tablet contains paracetamol. It is essential to read the contents of the medication you intend to take very carefully. Do not take paracetamol with another 'combination' drug which also contains paracetamol, since the possibility of accidentally over-dosing and causing liver or kidney damage is dramatically increased. Combination drugs can be helpful in reducing the number of tablets that need to be taken.

Co-codamol is a combination drug containing codeine and paracetamol. Codeine is a mild opiate analgesic that is similar to, but weaker than, morphine. When combined with paracetamol it can be extremely effective for moderate pain, but due to its codeine content, continued use can cause constipation. Although codeine itself can be habit-forming, this is very unlikely if the analgesia is used solely for the acute phase of your back pain.

Co-dydramol is another typical combination drug integrating paracetamol with dihydrocodeine. As its name suggests, dihydrocodeine is related to codeine, of similar potency and can also cause constipation if used long-term.

Co-proxamol – The efficacy and safety of drugs are always under review and another combination drug, co-proxamol, has recently had its licence withdrawn because of safety concerns, particularly due to its toxicity in overdose, which can affect respiration. It has also been discovered that the inclusion of dextropropoxyphene, a mild opiate analgesic, in this combination drug, is in any case no more effective than just taking paracetamol on its own.

Non-steroidal anti-inflammatory drugs

A separate group of drugs which are helpful for the relief of pain, stiffness and inflammation affecting muscles, bones and joints are non-steroidal anti-inflammatory drugs. They are frequently referred to as 'NSAIDs'. They are called 'non-steroidal' to distinguish them from corticosteroids, which are prescription-only medications used by medical practitioners to combat inflammation in specific medical conditions.

NSAIDs work by blocking the production of prostaglandins, which are the chemicals released by the body at the site of an injury and which produce inflammation and swelling. These drugs are usually effective within an hour and relieve pain by reducing the pressure caused by the inflammation. Generally they are very safe and effective drugs, but just occasionally, as they are rapidly absorbed by the digestive system, there is a slight risk to some people of their causing bleeding in the stomach or duodenum. They are therefore not recommended for people known to suffer from peptic ulcers. Most NSAIDS should not be taken during pregnancy and caution is advised for those people suffering from liver, kidney or blood clotting disorders. Asthma sufferers should also cease taking this group of drugs if there is any worsening of their condition, and seek medical advice.

Ibuprofen is a commonly available 'over the counter' NSAID medication, enormously effective for the reduction of pain, stiffness and inflammation. It has fewer side effects than many other non-steroidals and can be taken together with paracetamol if additional pain relief is required as the two drugs follow different 'pathways' in the body. Although ibuprofen is considered the gentlest of the non-steroidal drugs, many people are sensitive to this medication – for example, experiencing diarrhoea – and caution is recommended. Ibuprofen is also available as a gel or cream, which can be rubbed into the skin at the area of pain. It should not be used in this way, however, at the same time as taking the drug in tablet form as the overall intake of the drug is increased and could result in overdose.

Diclofenac is another extremely effective anti-inflammatory drug but is generally available by medical prescription only. Like ibuprofen, however, it is also available as an 'over the counter' gel. Rubbed into the painful area, it is highly beneficial but again, should not be used simultaneously with diclofenac in tablet form.

Muscle relaxants

There is yet one more group of drugs often prescribed by doctors. These are muscle relaxants. When muscle spasm is severe, many doctors now also prescribe a muscle relaxant in addition to analgesia to help provide relief during the initial acute phase. The involuntary, painful contraction of a muscle, or group of muscles, can make it almost impossible to straighten your back. The longer this severe spasm lasts, the greater the delay in relieving the pain and getting rest, both of which are essential components of the recovery process.

Muscle relaxant drugs work by damping down the nerve signals from the brain to the spinal cord which cause the muscles to contract. By interfering in this way, stiffness is reduced, allowing greater mobility. By their very nature, muscle relaxants can cause drowsiness, especially at the beginning of treatment. In addition, too high a dose can cause muscle weakness. For this reason, the dosage must be carefully adjusted to the individual patient by the doctor and instructions for the drug's administration followed with care.

Diazepam (valium) is probably the most commonly used muscle relaxant, although others are available to be prescribed at the discretion of the medical practitioner. For acute back pain and if spasm is severe, diazepam is usually prescribed for a short period (a few days) only or until the muscular contraction has subsided. For this reason, there is little likelihood of developing dependency on the drug, which can occur with long-term use.

Analgesia of whatever type and strength should always be taken regularly and in accordance with either the doctor's or manufacturer's instructions until you feel it is no longer required. Hopefully, after a short period of rest and suitable pain relief, the pain will begin to subside a little. Now is the time to start work on your muscles.

4. Movement and exercises

Muscles lose their strength very quickly. Only a few days of bed rest can leave you feeling generally weak and lethargic. It requires determination and sometimes hard work to fully regain mobility and fitness. For some, recovering from back pain may also inspire them to learn the benefits of good posture and techniques of safe moving and handling.

When the ache in your back is bad, even getting out of bed in the morning can be a painful experience. Such suffering at the beginning of the day may not only discourage remedial exercises but can also have a detrimental effect on your psychological approach to further activity.

The easiest way to get out of bed is to roll onto your side, facing the edge of the bed. Allow your feet and legs to drop towards the floor and simultaneously push your upper body into an upright sitting position, using both hands on the mattress. Standing up is then safer and less painful.

In the early stages of recovery activity should be very gentle and carried out in a warm and draught-free environment. The following are a few simple stretching movements, aimed at relieving the tension as well as the pain. It is, as already mentioned, a good idea to take appropriate analgesia about 20-30 minutes before-hand. Once these can be accomplished without recurrence of spasm or pain, progression to the exercises described in the next chapter will begin the programme of strengthening the back muscles and improving flexibility of your spine.

Early morning stretching

Step one

- Start by standing with your feet apart or sitting up as straight as you can on a dining-room chair.
- Placing your hands flat on your lower back you will be able to identify the actual area of stiffness and pain.
- Pull your tummy in towards your spine and, whilst taking slow, deep breaths, slowly and firmly massage the area with your fingers. This stimulation of the muscle fibres will help ease the stiffness, particularly if your back is crooked, and assist you in regaining your correct posture.

Step two

- Stand upright, lifting your ribs away from your abdomen.
- With your feet slightly apart (the width of your shoulders), place your opened hands on your lower back, on either side of your spine.
- Press your hands firmly into your back for added support and, whilst taking care to maintain your balance, raise your head slightly and lean backwards from your upper waist. You will feel your abdominal muscles take up the strain.
- As your spine arches a little backwards, your lower back muscles should be allowed to relax away from your normal posture.
- (One word of warning – do not be tempted to lean too far back so as to lose balance. It is better to hold a modest stance for several seconds than to over-stretch.)

Step 3

- Lie on your back (this can be done in bed or on the floor) and raise your knees so that your feet are flat on the surface on which you are lying.

- Pull your navel in as though you want it to touch your spine.
- Let your arms extend outwards into a downward 'V' shape and take in a slow, deep breath.
- As you let the breath out, gently twist from the waist to the right so that your knees lean over towards the floor.
- Try to hold this position for the count of five and then on an outward breath, bring your knees back up, returning to your original position.
- Repeat this on the left side.

Tips to help you stretch and warm up safely

- It is possible that the pain is not central, but more to one side than the other. In this case, exercise is likely to be more painful on that side and therefore the movement achieved will be unequal. Don't worry about this or concentrate your efforts only on the painful side. Continue to carry out all the exercises to both sides alike. The fact that pain is more prevalent in one area does not mean that all the associated muscles and ligaments do not need to benefit from these relaxation methods.
- As frustrating as back pain is, don't go beyond that which is comfortable. If an activity hurts, stop straight away. Repeat your breathing exercises, massage the area with strong circular movements and rest. Wait until you feel able to try it again.
- Bear in mind that it is not easy when the discomfort of back pain is gnawing away at you to consciously control your posture and carry out the exercises that relieve the problem. But when the pain disappears, so can the incentive to maintain the good work ... until the pain strikes again! And it may. Each episode of back pain increases the chance of it happening again unless the muscles are strengthened and posture improved.
- For those recovering from back pain and who normally enjoy regular energetic exercise, the question most often asked is, 'When can I start again?' The answer, of course, is individual to the sufferer. However, if you attempt vigorous exercise before full mobility and flexibility have been restored, it is likely that your movements will be unbalanced, putting strain on previously unaffected muscles.

Walking

Perhaps the most important exercise on the way to recovery from back pain is walking. Not just a wander down the garden, but as a specific exercise in its own right.

Walking correctly is half the battle. You may think that sounds daft, but over the years we develop all sorts of strange postures, including leaning forwards or backwards, eyes always focused on the ground, round-shouldered or allowing our feet to point outwards instead of in the direction of travel. In just the same way as it is important to learn the correct posture for standing and sitting, the way we walk is equally significant. The adjustments needed may only be slight, but the improved balance and deportment will relieve your back muscles of unnecessary strain, allowing them to relax into the movement. This will enable you to walk further, without the fatigue that perhaps made it an arduous task in the past.

Good, supportive shoes are the only equipment you need, apart from comfortable clothing appropriate for the weather and time of year. It is also a good idea to take a drink of water with you to avoid dehydration as you get warmed up.

To start with, set yourself a realistic route of, say, a mile. Don't set off on some route-march across rough, uneven ground. Not only will you become tired; the jarring pace over irregular terrain will further stress your tense muscles and have the opposite effect to that desired. Start slowly, aware of your walking posture, and work up to an energetic pace that gets you slightly out of breath. As you become fitter and your back pain recedes, increase the distance and range of your walks.

The stimulation to your cardio-vascular system will not only be good for your heart and lungs, but will increase the blood supply carrying oxygen to your muscles. As the oxygen is absorbed into the tissue spaces from the blood, it is exchanged for carbon dioxide and other waste products, including damaged cells from the site of inflammation which are then removed from the area.

Walking, of course, is free and can usually be fitted in to your normal daily routine. It is also an activity that can be enjoyed in the company of others. Whether you choose to walk with family or friends, or join a ramblers' association (these generally cater for all ages and levels of fitness), talking with others will not only enable you to walk greater distances without consciously being aware of it, but bring a level of enjoyment to an exercise programme, not possible with many other therapies.

Swimming and water treatments

Swimming is widely recognised as being the best complete aerobic exercise. Supported by the pressure of the water, every muscle and joint can be stretched and stimulated smoothly without the strain or jarring associated with, say, running. The advantages for sufferers of back pain are obvious. Weightlessness provides a freedom for uninhibited movement that is not possible in any other exercise regimen. Whilst it is not advisable to swim if muscle spasm is present, once you are through that, steady rhythmic strokes will be of enormous benefit, not just to your back but to your overall fitness.

Whether or not you are a competent swimmer, the buoyancy of deep water, even while holding onto the side of a swimming pool, is a great way to exercise your leg and back muscles. If excessive weight is also a problem, water exercises and swimming are of enormous benefit, since tense and painful muscles can achieve improved suppleness without excessive resistance whilst burning up fat at the same time. It is estimated that approximately 150 calories can be burned off in half an hour this way. Yet another advantage is that some facilities can be relatively inexpensive- and this form of exercise can often be fitted into your normal daily activities without the discipline of appointment times to keep. Swimming is also an exercise that can be shared with friends or relatives who can both support and encourage you as you regain your fitness. As a social activity it can be a lot of fun.

Following back pain, the crawl or back stroke are the most beneficial strokes. This is because with both movements the head can be kept in straight alignment to the rest of the spine. With the breast stroke, if your head is constantly held above the level of the water, strain can be put upon your neck and shoulder muscles and your back can become arched, creating an unnatural posture which may be uncomfortable. If, however, this is your preferred style and the one you feel safest with, it might help to purchase a pair of swimming goggles so that you are not so reluctant to lower your head as you stretch forwards at the beginning of each stroke.

There are many other forms of water treatment, including water massage and water aerobic classes. There are also floatation and therapeutic baths with hot water, some using copious amounts of Epsom salts to improve buoyancy, and in some cases, seaweed or sea minerals, all of which aim to provide weightless relaxation to relieve tension and discomfort.

Jogging

Jogging, or running, by its very nature, can subject the body, and in particular the back, to considerable jarring, especially if the running is predominantly on hard surfaces, such as concrete. If this is an activity you have previously enjoyed and provided you are comfortable to do so, a short distance of very slow running will not cause harm and may indeed help to warm and relax your muscles.

The three vital elements of running are **posture** (yes, that again), **correct footwear** and technique. If you've ever been an observer or participant in a marathon run, you will be aware that there are hundreds of different styles of jogging. Poor **technique** is the cause of much lower back pain. Pounding the ground, particularly when beginning to tire, causes shock waves which travel up from the feet to the hips and spine.

Posture – It is important to run effectively without distorting your posture, which may overstretch or overload your back muscles. Throughout the exercise, your body must be aligned from the shoulders, through to the hips and down to the forefoot which is touching the ground.

Running shoes – The type of shoes worn for running is extremely important. Running in old, poorly fitted trainers can in itself cause low back pain. It is a good idea, when purchasing a pair of running shoes, to take along your old ones to a shop specialising in sportswear so that the fitter can assess the way the shoes have worn. In this way any abnormal wearing of the sole can be corrected, sometimes by inserting an insole, to slightly adjust the way the weight is supported when your foot touches the ground.

Technique – Try to stay light on your feet, perhaps taking slightly shorter strides in order to keep a good, upright posture. Run with a heel to toe action, through the whole of the foot. Be relaxed, allow your shoulders to drop and concentrate more on a light, comfortable stride and less on covering the ground quickly. With your forearms raised, use the swing of your arms to aid your momentum and keep your upper body elevated from your waist. Avoid leaning too far forward. This can cause you to extend your landing foot too far in front, which results in the lower back adopting a rotating movement with each stride which will eventually lead to your back muscles becoming tight and painful.

Running on grass or a treadmill will help to reduce the jarring impact which can be caused by concrete pavements.

Tips to help you run safely

- Always do some warming-up and stretching exercises before you begin your run.
- Don't forget to repeat your warm-up exercises and stretches at the end of your run to help relieve any tension which may have built up in your muscles.
- Bear in mind that running up or down hills requires postural changes which will put greater stress on your back muscles and joints. It is therefore better to keep to level running until your general fitness is improved and back pain completely eliminated.
- Treadmills are a good way of reducing the impact of running. Their use not only removes the inclination to 'push forwards' with each stride, but has the advantage that you can stop immediately if you start to feel pain.
- As with all exercises, if jogging causes any pain, stop. Return to a vigorous walk and try jogging another time.

Chapter 12

Exercises to strengthen back muscles

Unfortunately, there is no quick 'fix' for back pain. Recovery is mostly down to gentle exercise. For many people, the very word 'exercise' conjures up images of school-day physical education classes, being hot, sweaty and out of breath. This might inspire athletes but certainly not those whose only ambition is to relieve nagging pain, get back to normal living and strengthen the muscles that have been injured so that the problem doesn't happen again.

When every tiny movement takes your breath away and grips your back like an invisible vice, the last thing you may want to think about is exercise. However, the sooner movement and gentle mobility can be re-introduced, the quicker the recovery – honestly! We're not talking here about gymnastics, but slow, gentle stretching movements which can both aid the relaxation of muscles and improve the suppleness of joints. No exercise should ever be painful. If it hurts, stop. Rest awhile and try again, paying particular attention to assessing the accuracy and precision of each movement. Exercise should never aggravate or increase pain. If there are no early signs of improvement it is essential that you see a doctor for a full examination to eliminate the possibility of any other underlying medical condition. As muscle stiffness appears to improve, you may, of course, be keen to get started, and who can blame you? For some, there is a great temptation, when making the commitment to carry out an exercise or fitness regimen, to want to do too much, too soon. This type of exercise, however, should never be embarked upon with a sudden great rush of enthusiasm and vigour or carried out to excess. Without wishing to dampen your enthusiasm, it is important to point out that slow, con-sistent progression is the way to strengthen muscles and restore good flexibility. Launching into an over-ambitious programme from the start will inevitably cause further pain and may put you off altogether. Consider carefully the advice given in chapter 11 relating to the commencement of exercises and progress slowly.

Do not exercise immediately after eating a meal. Exercises should not be hurried, so try to find opportunities during the day when you are not likely to be interrupted. If back pain and stiffness are present, it is better to carry out frequent, short sessions of, say, 10 to 15 minutes at a time, rather than a prolonged session once a day. Even in the busiest of households, it should be possible to make use of opportunities, perhaps when the children are at school or baby is sleeping, or maybe while the family is watching the television.

Always wear loose, comfortable clothing, such as a tee-shirt and slacks. Tight jeans and belts not only restrict your movements but will make them less effective.

Take it steady to start with, introducing only gentle stretching exercises. A good plan is to start with two of the easier exercises and carry them out every couple of hours with sensitivity and without strain. After a day or two, exchange one of the exercises for a different, slightly more advanced one, but always keeping your sessions to about 10 minutes. This way the muscles are flexed frequently but able to relax in between so that you are not left feeling tired and aching from excessive effort. Progression is up to you. As strength and fitness return, extend the range of physical activities.

Remember too that re-training your body to maintain correct posture for all movements is essential in reducing the likelihood of a recurrence of back pain.

The exercises described here have originated from several sources. Some may be recognisable as adaptations of Pilates or Yoga movements, whilst others have been recommended by physiotherapists or orthopaedic doctors. Based on this wide practical experience, all have been practised and found to be hugely beneficial by the author of this book in her own success in overcoming back pain. Below are two of examples of where this approach has been successful for others:

- **Eileen**, 34, slipped, but without falling, on ice outside her home when leaving to escort her children to school. In doing so, she wrenched the muscles in her lower back and, although she bravely struggled on, by the time she returned home the spasm in her back was intolerable. Analgesia, the application of hot and cold compresses to the painful area, and gentle exercises ensured she was able to walk pain-free within a few days.
- **Barry**, 58, a lorry driver, had been dogged for years by intermittent sciatic pain due to the constant vibration on long-distance journeys. Regular

stretching exercises, including the 'knee to chest' stretch (described later in this chapter) relieved the pressure on his sciatic nerve, and using a lumbar support on the driver's seat has prevented the return of his pain.

Stretches and active movements are divided into two sections below. The first exercises described are particularly beneficial for relieving tension and spasm following muscle strain. These basic stretches should be carried out until they can be done comfortably and without pain.

The second group of movements are intended to promote muscle development and control. By building on the postural improvement of your body and adding strength and flexibility to your muscles, the risk of further back strain will be greatly reduced.

Breathing

Whether or not back pain is present when you embark on a programme of exercise, there is one important element vital to the success and ease with which stretching and strengthening movements can be achieved. This is good effective breathing. Take a few moments to be quite still and breathe deeply and slowly. This will not only improve the oxygenation of your muscles, but will encourage you to relax, both mentally and physically. This will help relieve some of the tension that has built up from either a busy lifestyle or the constant tension of pain. Try to get into the habit of closing your eyes and very slowly inhaling and exhaling to your maximum lung capacity. Do this five times before and after each exercise session.

For each of the exercises described, it is important that you first take in a slow, deep breath and carry out the movement on the outward breath. The effort is therefore carried out as the diaphragm and chest muscles relax to expel the air and while the level of oxygen in the muscles is at its optimum. Taking an inward breath requires some tension of the muscles and this can make the movement less effective.

SECTION ONE – GENTLE MOVEMENTS

Wake-up stretches

There are various stretches that can be done first thing in the morning, before you even get out of bed.

- Lie on your back with one pillow placed under your head.

- As with all exercise postures or movements, remember to prepare for the action with five slow deep breaths.
- On the last expiration, pull your tummy in towards your back as though trying to make your navel touch your spine.
- Now reach as far as you can to the bottom of the bed with one pointed foot.
- Hold it there and count to five.
- Relax.
- Do the same stretch with the other foot.
- Repeat the sequence five times.
- Rotate both feet as though drawing circles with your toes. This is a good way to stimulate the circulation to your lower body before attempting to get out of bed.

Abdominal muscle warm-up

One of the first and most important exercises is aimed at strengthening your abdominal muscles. Developing the good habit of always involving your abdominal muscles in all your daily activities will ensure that your back is given enormously improved support and the risk of injury is dramatically reduced. The following exercise can be done as a floor exercise or even carried out with your back against a wall. Whichever method you use, this is a good exercise with which to begin a work-out programme, but can also be practised in any opportune moment during a busy day.

Method one
- If using the floor, lie on your back with knees raised and feet flat on the ground.
- Tilt your pelvis so that the whole of your lower spine is touching the floor.
- Take in a slow, deep breath and as you exhale, imagine a cord pulling your navel down towards your spine.
- Hold the position to a count of five and repeat it 10 times.

Method two
If you do not feel ready to try exercising on the floor:
- Stand as tall as you can with your back against the wall.

- Tuck your bottom in so that there is no gap between your lower spine and the wall.
- As you exhale a deep breath, pull your navel in towards your spine and hold it to a count of five.
- Repeat this 10 times.

Belly twist

This movement can be done either whilst lying on a bed or on a mat on the floor.

- Lie on your back and pull your tummy in, pressing your back down so that the natural curve of your spine is flattened onto the bed / floor.
- Raise your knees so that your feet are flat on the mattress or floor.
- Outstretch both arms, level with your shoulders.
- As you expel your breath, allow your knees to gently rest down to the right, keeping your shoulders and arms flat on the bed.
- Relax and count to five.
- Breathe in and again, as you expel the air, return your knees to their upright position.
- Carry out the action to the left side and repeat this five times.

This movement helps to release tension caused by recent spasm while the muscles are still warm from the bed (see Figure 12.1).

Figure 12.1 Belly twist.

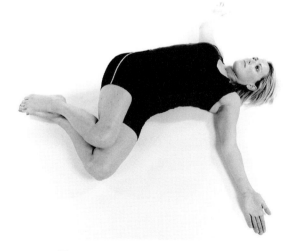

Cat stretches

One of the most effective exercises for both stretching and relieving tension in the back is the 'cat stretch'. Variations of this movement can be found in many complementary therapies. Performed slowly, it will improve the flexibility of your spine and muscles, even when a little back stiffness is present. If any strain is felt, however, you should stop immediately and try it again another time.

As its name suggests, the pose for this exercise imitates the waking stretch of feline animals.

- Kneel on the floor with your knees directly beneath and the same width apart as your hips.
- Place your hands flat on the floor directly under your shoulders and make your back as straight as you can.
- Look at the floor so that your head is held in line with your spine. There should be no strain on your neck. Your overall position should resemble a flat table.
- Take a steady breath in.
- Pull your navel in towards your spine and as you exhale, slowly lift your back into an arch, allowing your head to fall down until your ears touch the inside of your arms. The whole length of your spine should be stretched in an arch, but without undue strain (see Figure 12.2).
- Now, reverse the stretch by lifting your head so that you can look forwards, simultaneously lowering your back until it arches downwards as far as you can comfortably manage.
- Hold each pose to a count of five before relaxing, and repeat both movements 10 times (see Figure 12.3).

Child's pose

Another good stretching exercise, as recommended by Yoga therapists, is the 'child's pose'. This is another movement which can be done on a bed if getting down to and up from the floor is difficult.

This exercise is aimed at stretching the spine so that the vertebrae are opened up along its entire length, but without carrying the weight of the body. It should be a relaxing pose and without strain, although to start with existing stiffness may make the optimum position difficult to achieve. Don't worry – it will become

Figure 12.2 Cat stretches – arched with lowered head.

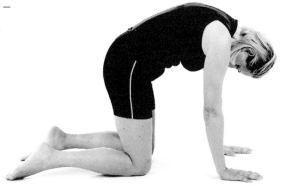

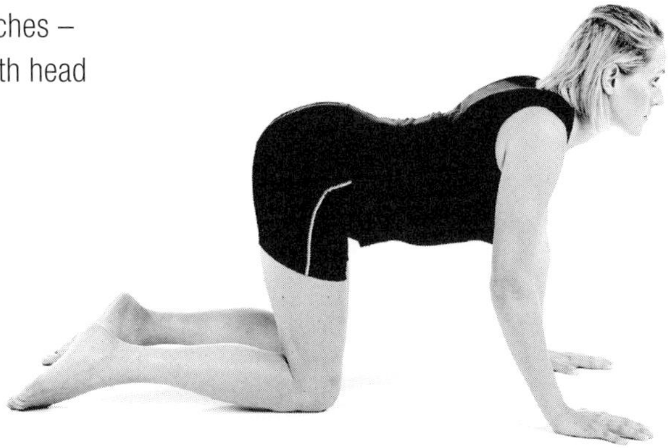

Figure 12.3 Cat stretches – arched downwards with head raised.

easier as your back becomes more flexible.

- Kneel on the bed or floor and sit back onto your heels.
- Open your knees by pointing them slightly out to the sides.
- Now reach forwards with your hands on the floor in front of you. The gap between your knees should help you to condense your shape, stretching the whole of your back (without becoming hunched) whilst pushing your hands before you as far as you can.
- Look down towards the floor so that your neck is not arched. You may even be able to touch the floor with your forehead, although this may not be possible to start with.

- One by one, take your arms back and rest them on the ground beside your legs with the palms of your hands facing uppermost.
- Relax. Breathe slowly and deeply for as long as you feel comfortable to hold this position (see Figure 12.4)
- Bring your arms forward again and use them to push you back upright, sitting well back onto your heels as you do so.

Knee to chest

This stretching exercise is excellent for the *piriformis* muscle, which lies deep inside the buttock and is occasionally responsible for sciatic pain.

- Lie on your back with both legs stretched out together.
- Pull up one leg towards your chest and hold it in position just below the knee with the hand on that same side of your body.
- Now, replace that hand with the other one.
- Keep your shoulders flat on the floor.
- As you expel a large breath, gently pull the knee across your body until you feel the stretch in your buttock.
- Hold this position for a count of five before returning your knee to its upright position.
- Repeat this same stretch two or three times before resting your leg down.
- Now carry out the same movement using the other leg, reversing the actions (see Figure 12.5).

SECTION TWO – MORE ADVANCED MOVEMENTS

Twisted pose

This is a variation on the 'belly twist' movement, which will increase the stretch. It is a more advanced move which engages the lower back, abdominal and buttock muscles.

- Lie flat on the floor with arms extended to the sides at shoulder height.
- Turn your head to the right; as you exhale, lift your right leg over the left one as far as you can and rest your knee on the floor at right angles to your hip.
- Return to your start position and repeat on the other side (see Figure 12.6).

Figure 12.4 Child's pose.

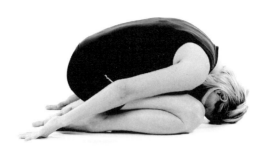

Figure 12.5 Knee to chest stretch – right hand pulls left leg gently across body.

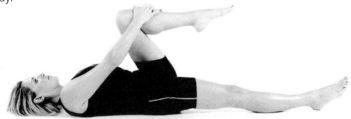

Figure 12.6 Twisted pose – knee rests on floor at right angles to hip.

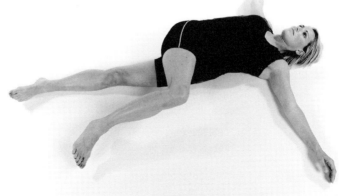

Figure 12.7 Extended cat
stretches.

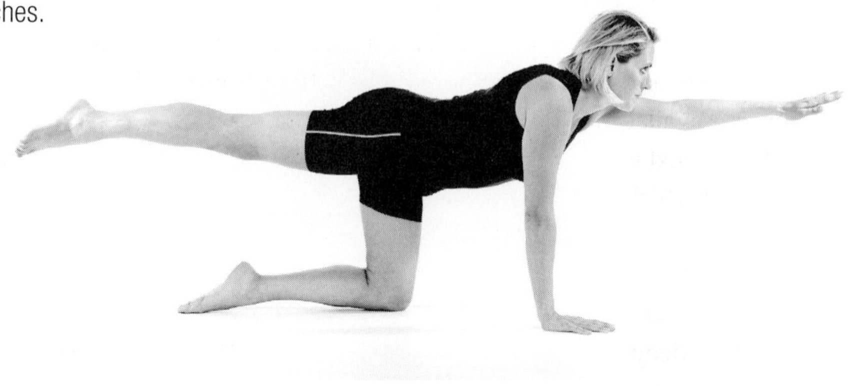

Extended cat stretches

A rather more advanced variation on the previously described 'cat stretch' exercises stems from the same basic pose.

- Kneel with your knees directly beneath your hips and your hands flat on the floor beneath your shoulders.
- Keep your back straight and your head in line, so that you again take the shape of a table.
- Breathe in and pull your navel in towards your spine.
- As you exhale, stretch your right leg out behind you so that it is level with your spine.
- Point your toes.
- Now reach forwards with your left hand at shoulder height, but keeping your head facing downwards or eyes focused no higher than the fingertips of your elevated arm so as not to strain your neck.
- Hold this position for a count of 10 before slowly returning your knee to the floor.
- Now do the same with the opposite leg and arm.

Provided the exercise causes no discomfort, repeat it 10 times (see Figure 12.7).

Side stretches

This exercise, although simple in its concept, may be a difficult one to achieve if you are suffering back pain which is predominantly on one side. The aim is to flex the spine in a sideways arch by stretching the supportive muscles in order to release tension. Since it involves a stance seldom used in daily living, it may take practice over a period of time in order to achieve a significant bend, but it nevertheless helps to lengthen the spinal column. It can be helpful to use a full-length mirror, if you have one available, to enable you to check that your alignment is correct.

- Stand next to, and with one hand hold the back of, a chair or other sturdy object which is about waist height.
- With your feet hip width apart, stand tall and pull your navel in towards your spine.
- Relax your shoulders.
- Take a deep breath in and, as you then exhale, lift your outer arm away from your body to the side and continue up until it is above your head.
- As far as you can comfortably do so, reach past your head until your spine and upper body bend sideways towards the chair.
- Be careful not to twist or even slightly lean forward or the benefit of the stretch will be lost and your posture will be compromised (see Figure 12.8).

Figure 12.8 Side stretches – note, no twisting or leaning forward.

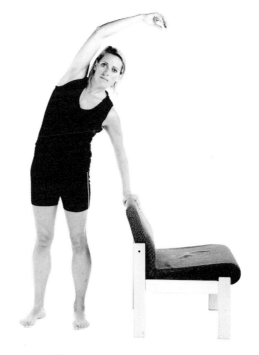

- Turn to face the other way and repeat the stretch on the other side.

To start with, if one side is stiff from injury, you may not achieve an equal bend to each side. Over time, and as your stiffness subsides, you will be able to judge your improvement as the sideways arch increases and becomes more evenly matched.

Side leg raises

Although this exercise is carried out while lying on your side, it is especially good for improving the strength of both your abdominal muscles and your buttocks. Don't forget that the buttocks are a huge muscle mass and a valuable contributor to both posture and strength.

This is not a suitable movement to be carried out on your bed as the softness of the mattress will give insufficient support, allowing your body to bend in the middle.

- To start with, lie on your side in a long straight line and with the underarm on the extended above your head.
- Let your head rest on the upper part of this arm.
- Keep your knees and ankles together, with your legs straight.
- As you breathe out, pull your navel inwards, slightly tilt your pelvis forwards so that it slightly increases the arch of your back. Lift your upper-most leg a few inches and hold it there.
- Count to five before lowering the leg.
- Repeat the movement five times.
- Turn onto your other side and repeat the movement, raising the other leg in the same way.

This movement can be further advanced by lifting both legs together about two inches from the floor and holding the position to a count of five (see Figure 12.9).

As your lower back and abdomen become stronger, you will be able to maintain this position, perhaps to the count of 10, but to start with just gently raise and lower your legs without causing undue strain.

Free-fall pose

This is an advanced exercise which can greatly improve the strength of your back muscles but should not be attempted until all signs of back pain have gone. If this

Figure 12.9 Side leg raises.

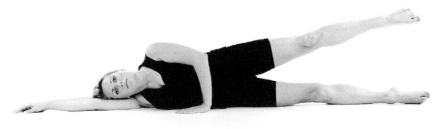

Figure 12.10 Free-fall pose.

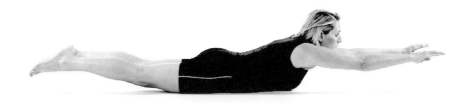

movement causes pain or is too difficult, stop immediately.

The aim is to contract the back muscles in order to pull the spine into a backward arch, thus pulling the upper torso and legs upwards, while the floor supports the bulk of the body's weight.

- Lie prone (face down) on the floor or mat with your arms extended in front.
- Take a deep, controlled breath in, and as you then slowly exhale, lift your arms and feet an inch or two from the floor.
- Look forwards and hold the position for a count of five.
- Then lower your limbs and relax.
- Do not strain (see Figure 12.10).

Abdominal pull-ups

This advanced exercise is very good for strengthening the abdominal muscles, but should be executed with great care to avoid putting unnecessary strain on

Figure 12.11 Abdominal pull-ups – note the whole back must be in contact with the floor.

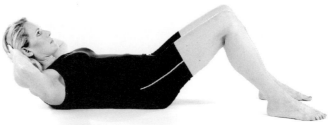

your back.

- Lie on your back, with your knees raised and your feet pressed firmly on the floor.
- Clasp your hands behind your head.
- Pull your navel in towards your spine and push your feet against the resistance of the floor so that the whole of your back is in contact with the floor. This preparation position is **vital** in order to prevent the normal curvature of your spine taking the strain.
- Now, as you exhale, raise your head and shoulders 5-10 centimetres from the ground and lower again immediately.
- The movement is small and can be repeated 10-15 times or until you feel your tummy muscles begin to pull (see Figure 12.11).
- This toning exercise is also good for those trying to lose weight and working towards a flatter tummy.

Key points

- To recover from back pain, gentle movement should be started as soon as possible.

- But do not do too much too soon.

- Frequent short sessions will be more effective than one long session.

- Aim for slow but consistent progression.

- Start with gentle stretching exercises.

- Build up gradually to muscle-strengthening exercises.

- Effective and controlled breathing is essential.

- No exercise should ever be painful; if it is, STOP!

Chapter 13

Orthodox and medical treatments

There are very many different therapies and medical treatments associated with back pain. From straight-forward exercise programmes through to invasive spinal surgery, their aim is to relieve the suffering that results from this disabling condition.

It can be confusing, with such a diverse range of treatments available, to understand what each of them means and what is involved. It is important to remember that any form of medical treatment must be appropriate to the individual needs of the patient and will only be recommended as the result of a professional consultation with those who specialise in resolving back problems.

Those treatments associated with the medical profession are described briefly below so that you will have an understanding of what the options are and what is being recommended if a specialist prescribes one of these alternatives for you. They are not listed in order of suitability, benefit or recommendation, but purely in order of those which are likely to be most familiar to you or about which you may have heard, starting with the least intrusive.

Physiotherapy

For many people, physiotherapy is perhaps the most commonly known restorative treatment. As part of orthodox medical treatment, it is a service provided within hospitals and general practices for those recovering from operations or certain medical conditions. It is also widely used within professional sports organisations, many of which employ their own physiotherapists to ensure the high fitness standards required in today's sporting arena. However, physiotherapists are involved in very many different aspects of health and wellbeing. Working with clients of all ages, they aim to re-establish mobility and prevent further injury in order to restore active independence where required.

We tend to think of physiotherapy as a modern treatment, used only as a supplement to orthodox medicine, but its origins go back as far as 460 BC, when manual therapy, hydrotherapy and massage are believed to have been used by the well-known physician Hippocrates. However, it was not until 1813 that Per Henrik Ling, who founded the Royal Institute of Gymnastics in Sweden, and whose techniques for massage, manipulation and exercise were officially recognised by Sweden's National Board of Health and Welfare, formed the principles on which today's profession is underpinned. Great Britain, New Zealand and USA soon developed schools of physiotherapy (or 'physical therapy') and increasing popularity has since seen it advance throughout the world.

The early 20th century saw enormous developments in the scope and range of rehabilitation through the use of exercise, massage and traction. Physical function restored to injured soldiers during the First World War demonstrated the benefits of the therapy.

Today, physiotherapists are qualified practitioners, able to administer many different types of treatment, including manipulation, ultrasound and interferential (electrical current) therapy, hydrotherapy and acupuncture, as well as passive and active exercises to relieve pain and stiffness. All the treatments are based upon well-researched and approved techniques and are chosen according to the individual needs of each client.

As with other therapies, an initial extensive assessment is carried out both to identify problems and to establish an appropriate programme of treatment which will achieve the best possible outcome. The assessment itself uses a holistic approach, taking into consideration not just physical mobility and weaknesses, but medical history, and psychological, social and cultural factors, in order to gain a true overall picture of the problem.

A large part of physiotherapists' work includes treating pain and immobility due to back injuries. Some physiotherapists specialise in particular aspects of their profession, choosing to concentrate on disorders of the musculoskeletal system, including back and spinal conditions. Many of these work alongside orthopaedic surgeons within a hospital setting. All use a range of 'hands on' techniques in the treatment of back pain, such as massage, manipulation, heat, cold, electric current and remedial exercises in order to restore mobility and promote healing. They also recommend appropriate exercises to be continued at home to encourage active rehabilitation. Education is also important. Advice, exercise routines which may be continued at home and, in some cases, lifestyle changes, are all aimed at both preventing a recurrence of the problem and equipping the individual to continue an active and independent life.

In most countries, physiotherapists are easily available, although there can sometimes be a considerable wait for treatment due to the huge demand for their services. They can sometimes be sourced in doctors' surgeries, leisure centres and health centres, and are even provided by some of the larger companies. Although some health service providers may offer physiotherapy without charge, private practices will obviously charge according to the length, type and frequency of the treatment required. The provision of physiotherapy by private health insurance companies is determined by the individual policy.

As recognised professional practitioners, physiotherapists have undergone an intensive three–four year degree course, are governed by a Professional Code of Conduct and are covered by professional liability insurance. As with all therapies, it is important to ensure that the appropriate letters of qualification are shown after their name (that is, 'SRP' – State Registered Physiotherapist – or 'MCSP' – Member of the Chartered Society of Physiotherapy) and that they are registered with the governing body.

Tens machines

'TENS' stands for transcutaneous electrical nerve stimulation. That sounds complicated, but basically it means stimulating the body's own natural defence against pain by sending a very small electrical current through the skin. A gentle sensation of tingling or pins and needles, which is not unpleasant, can be felt in the area being treated. This is based on the 'gate theory of pain' developed by Patrick Wall and Ron Melzack in the 1960s to explain why thoughts and emotions affect the perception of pain.

The Tens machine works by giving a strong sensory signal to those nerves located in the area of the pain that normally identify touch and temperature. This stimulus replaces the pain signal, which is being sent up the spine to the brain, substituting it with a gentle tingling feeling in the area affected. This is known professionally as the 'pain gate', which can be opened or closed to let pain through.

Two small self-adhesive patches, or electrodes, are linked to the Tens machine by fine cables. The machines themselves vary slightly in size, but are generally not much bigger than a mobile phone and can be easily attached to a belt or placed in a pocket. The equipment is battery operated, with easy-to-use buttons which control both the intensity of the impulses and the mode, or programme (see below) desired. The two electrodes are attached to the skin and placed a short distance apart. Generally, most benefit is experienced when one electrode is positioned where the pain is greatest and the other over the spine and slightly higher than the painful area. However, if this combined position fails to give adequate pain relief, the manufacturers of Tens machines also suggest trying alternative sites until maximum benefit is felt.

There are two main modes of operation to choose between – 'pain gate mode' and 'low pulse rate mode'. In the 'pain gate mode', where the Tens machine emits a pulse rate of 110 Hz, relief is best provided while the machine is switched on; its longer-term effect may diminish after one to two hours. After a break of an hour you can try again. It is safe to use the Tens machine several times a day.

The main alternative programme sets the machine to a 'low pulse rate' of between 4 and 10 Hz. At this setting, the Tens causes the body to release endorphins, which are the body's own pain-relieving substances and which act in the same way as morphine. In this mode, relief builds up over 30 to 40 minutes and can provide further pain relief for as much as four hours. The Tens machine will then need to be applied again as pain returns.

Other programmes suggested by the manufacturers offer slight variations on these same principles, so experimentation using the different settings and strengths is well worth trying in order to ensure maximum benefit for you.

In rare cases, sensitivity to the electrodes may cause skin irritation, in which case the Tens should be discontinued and professional medical advice sought.

Tens machines are an easy, non-invasive method of pain relief with no known side effects, apart from the possible skin irritation just mentioned. Their use is widely recommended by hospital pain services and general practitioners as a good method of managing pain. For those individuals who prefer to limit the amount of oral analgesic medication they consume, these compact machines can offer a realistic alternative. They are widely available for purchase through most pharmaceutical outlets at prices ranging from £20 to £80. However, before making such a purchase, it is strongly recommended that you obtain a machine on trial first, either from your local doctor or hospital, to ascertain that it does indeed provide adequate pain relief in a way suitable for you as an individual.

It is important to remember, of course, that this is only a method of controlling pain and not a 'cure' for a bad back. However, periods of pain relief create the ideal opportunities in which to stretch and exercise the back muscles to improve both strength and mobility.

Injections

Facet joint injections

Many hospitals now provide pain clinics where doctors and nurses who have trained particularly in the treatment of chronic and post-surgical pain offer specialised treatment including injections for back pain. Most people are referred to the pain clinic by an orthopaedic surgeon or other consultant when more conservative methods have proved ineffective or surgical intervention is deemed to be unsuitable. One treatment offered in this context is injections in the back, from which some people find they may get considerable benefit.

One such type of injection which your pain specialist may advise for some patients with back pain is the facet joint injection (also called 'facet joint block'). The facet joints are located on the back of the spine on each side of the vertebrae where it overlaps the adjacent vertebrae (see Figure 13.1).

As part of the 'knobbly' protrusions at the back of the vertebrae, they determine the amount of movement that the spine can achieve. They also provide stability and give the spine the ability to bend and twist. However, a sharp jolt or sudden twisting movement can cause this part of the vertebrae to become bruised. Inflammation to these joints can irritate or squeeze the adjacent nerves, resulting in back pain and affecting the area supplied by that nerve.

In a facet joint injection, a combination of numbing local anaesthetic and anti-inflammatory steroid is injected into the joint using a thin needle. Depending on the location and extent of the pain, one or more joints may be injected. If the pain

Figure 13.1 Facet joints and how they can give rise to problems.

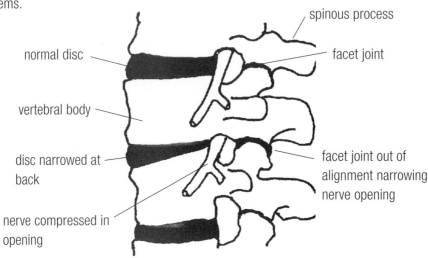

spinous process

normal disc

facet joint

vertebral body

disc narrowed at back

facet joint out of alignment narrowing nerve opening

nerve compressed in opening

subsides after the injection, this suggests that the injected facet joints are indeed the source of the trouble. After a successful injection the pain will disappear immediately and this will last for a few hours until the effect of the local anaesthetic wears off. It usually takes 5–7 days for the anti-inflammatory effect of the steroid to kick in and alleviate the pain, but relief from these injections can last from several days to several months.

If the suspected source of pain is from the **sacroiliac joints**, they may also be injected at the same time. The sacroiliac (or 'SI') joint is a large joint between the sacrum (the five fused vertebrae at the base of the spine which form part of the pelvic basin) and the ilium (the large flaring structure which forms the hipbone) of the pelvis. It is joined together by strong ligaments. The human body has two sacroiliac joints, one on the left and one on the right (see Figure 13.2).

Facet joint injections are performed under a local anaesthetic, although some patients may need sedation. The procedure is performed under fluoroscopic X-ray guidance that helps correct placement of the injection(s).

It is vital to recognise that the pain relief from such injections should not replace the need for a proper exercise programme to strengthen the back muscles. Facet joint injections ideally should be used as a method of allowing patients to

Figure 13.2 The position of the sacroiliac joints.

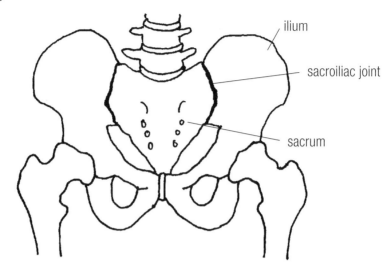

ilium

sacroiliac joint

sacrum

perform other forms of conservative treatment, such as physical exercise, Yoga, Pilates and stretching and bending, rather than a stand-alone treatment.

If the steroid injections provide good but temporary relief from the pain, the pain specialist may recommend a **radiofrequency neurotomy** (sometimes referred to as 'denervation' or 'rhizotomy' treatment). The purpose of this is to provide longer-lasting pain relief by disabling the sensory nerve that carries pain to the brain from the facet joint and/or sacroiliac joint.

In this injection procedure, a needle with a probe is inserted near the nerve. Once the sensory nerve has been identified, it is numbed with local anaesthetic and then the probe is heated with radio frequency waves. This deadens the sensory nerve connected to the joints and prevents the pain signals from getting to the brain.

Success rates for this procedure vary, but typically about 30–50% of patients undergoing this treatment may experience significant facet, or sacroiliac, joint pain relief. Of the remainder, about 50% will get some pain relief for a shorter period. However, some patients may not experience any relief. This is a safe procedure with few side effects, provided it is carried out by highly skilled medical professionals, such as anaesthetists, and performed under sterile conditions. The injection itself can sometimes be a little uncomfortable and, as said earlier, a little sedation may make the procedure more acceptable.

If effective, the 'neurotomy' (literally, division of the nerve) should provide relief from facet or sacroiliac joint pain for an average of 9–14 months and sometimes longer. After this period of time, however, the nerve will regenerate and the facet or sacroiliac joint pain may return; the procedure could then be repeated.

Epidural injections

Epidural injections are a relatively modern and, now, well-recognised method of pain relief for those suffering from chronic lower back pain. A local anaesthetic together with an anti-inflammatory steroid medication are injected into the painful area between the vertebrae and the outer membrane of the spinal cord, which is called the epidural space (see Figure 13.3). Like facet joint injections, this treatment is sometimes tried when other non-invasive treatments have been unsuccessful and also for those for whom surgery is unsuitable. It is not an alternative to surgery and is unlikely to provide permanent pain relief, although repeated treatments can be enormously beneficial over a number of years.

Like facet joint injections, epidurals work by enveloping the nerves which convey the pain signals to the brain in a local anaesthetic and steroidal solution. In this way, the transmission of pain impulses to the cerebral cortex can be blocked and long-term relief of several months can often be experienced following one injection. Most people are familiar with epidurals for pain relief in childbirth and surgery. For these situations, of course, depending on the drugs used, the duration of the effect may be short-lived – just a few hours for childbirth and a few days for post-operative pain relief.

Unlike routine injections of vaccines, or local anaesthetics for simple external procedures such as suturing or dental work, an epidural injection must be carried out in a sterile environment. Just as with facet joint injections, the doctor will 'scrub up', wear sterile gloves, clean the patient's back with anti-septic solution and cover the site of the lower back with a specially designed drape which has an opening in its centre through which the procedure is done.

Initially a small amount of local anaesthetic drug is injected to numb the area to make the procedure more comfortable. This is followed by the insertion of the

Figure 13.3 Cross-section through the spine to show the epidural space – the site for epidural injections.

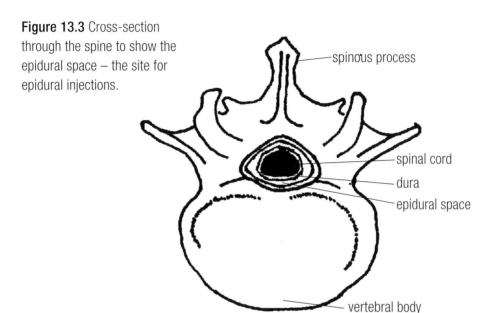

spinous process

spinal cord

dura

epidural space

vertebral body

epidural needle into the epidural space. Once the needle is in the space, the local anaesthetic and steroidal drug can be injected. Whilst the whole procedure is not particularly uncomfortable, it may take time and some patients are more at ease if a little sedation is given before the treatment starts.

Following a short rest of an hour or two, patients are usually allowed home. Due to the effect of the local anaesthetic drug, pain relief is usually immediate. However, it will generally last only a few hours. The steroidal drug takes much longer to be fully effective. This means that there is a short period of time, sometimes as long as 24 hours, between the wearing off of the local anaesthetic and the commencement of the longer-term pain relief provided by the steroids. At this stage, one might be forgiven for believing that the epidural has not worked, for not only will the original pain have returned, but the site of the injection may also feel a little sore. However, if the local anaesthetic did give good pain relief while it lasted, then the steroids should work too, since they were both injected into the same place.

For this reason, specific precautionary advice will be given before discharge from the hospital or clinic following these types of injection. Care must be taken when moving about during the first few hours following the injection as it can sometimes make patients' legs feel weak. The advice will likely include the avoidance of carrying hot drinks, taking great care when using stairs and generally to take it easy for the remainder of that day. Following a night's rest, mobility and strength should be back to normal.

Epidural injections, although very effective for most people, are seldom the 'cure' we would like them to be, since they only temporarily eliminate the pain. Two to three months is the average respite, although some can experience at least six months of pain-free mobility before the effect wears off. Everybody's experience is different.

The value that this method of treatment has for the sufferer is enormous. Without pain, the quality of sleep is improved, the need for oral analgesic pain-killers is reduced and almost normal daily activity can be resumed. The likelihood of depression is also reduced.

The downside of this treatment is its cost and availability. Research is on-going to evaluate the long-term effects of receiving medication in this way over many years, but thankfully to date major adverse results are rare.

Epidural injections should always be administered by a doctor, usually a trained anaesthetist who has specialised in this technique. Although a few family doctors with a professional interest in chronic pain have received appropriate training, generally referrals are made to chronic pain clinics incorporated within a hospital setting. Here the injections can be carried out under asepsis (a sterile procedure) and under the guidance, if needed, of an image intensifier (X-ray machine).

This invasive treatment is not appropriate for everyone with chronic back pain and a lengthy medical and physical examination will be required before it can be recommended. Private clinics also exist where this method of pain relief can be obtained but, of course, personal costs are involved.

Many sufferers, who previously could not get out of their homes due to severe back pain and disability, have benefited enormously from epidural injections by regaining their independence and social activities. Recent financial constraints, particularly in the UK, have caused a review of the provision of the specialised pain services within Britain's National Health Service. There is no doubt, however, that for those suffering chronic and debilitating pain, this treatment, although costly, has been proven to be hugely beneficial.

Spinal surgery

Surgery for back pain is generally a treatment of very last resort. It is not a quick fix, nor does it always result in complete success. For this reason several types of more conservative treatment should and will be tried first to resolve back pain before any recommendation is suggested for surgical intervention. These often include referrals to a physiotherapist, acupuncturist, pain specialist, chiropractor or a massage therapist.

The intricate work required, in the proximity of so important an area as the spine, is undertaken only by those experienced and highly skilled in this type of orthopaedic or neuro-surgery. The decision to embark upon such an operation is generally after a frank and informative discussion with the surgeon and after due consideration of his/her advice.

As with all wounds, as well as those resulting from surgical incision, healing involves the formation of scar tissue. In most cases this does not cause a problem, but for some people, excessive scar tissue can be created which will, over a period of time, re-establish the pressure on the very nerve that needed surgical treatment in the first place. This results in the reappearance of the back pain, and the subsequent likelihood of a full recovery is greatly reduced. Surgical operations of any kind carry a certain amount of risk and procedures carried out on the spine are no exception. Wound infection is probably the most likely complication, but bleeding and adverse reactions to anaesthesia can also be a problem. As previously stated, it is one of the last options available for those suffering from persistent back pain and should not be viewed as the ultimate 'cure'.

There are several specific surgical procedures, depending on the cause of the back problem. For most sufferers of unresolved back pain, the following (very brief) descriptions of operations are the most likely to be offered. Other procedures, not explained in this book, may be technically more appropriate for you but will depend on the individual circumstances and professional decision of the surgeon.

Discectomy, microdiscectomy, endoscopic discectomy and laser discectomy

Laser discectomy is the removal of a portion of an intervertebral disc where it has prolapsed and become squashed between two vertebrae. By excising the bulged portion, the pressure is released from the exiting nerve.

Foraminotomy

A foraminotomy is performed to relieve the symptoms of nerve root compression in cases where the foramen (opening in the bone through which a nerve passes) is being compressed by bone, disc, scar tissue or excessive ligament development and results in the nerve being pinched as it exits the spinal cord.

Laminectomy

A laminectomy is done to relieve pressure on the spinal cord itself. It is most commonly used to treat conditions such as spinal stenosis (narrowing of the spinal canal) and spondylolisthesis (a displacement of one vertebrae sliding over another). Depending on the amount of bone removed, this procedure may be done with a spinal fusion to prevent instability.

Spine fusion

Spine fusion is surgery that is done to eliminate motion between adjacent vertebrae. This may be carried out in order to treat a problem such as spondylolisthesis (a condition where one vertebra has slid forwards over another) or it may be done because of the extent of other surgery (such as a laminectomy – see above).

Spinal disc replacement

Spinal disc replacement is still a fairly new procedure and not yet commonplace. As its name suggests, the damaged intervertebral disc is removed and replaced by a synthetic prosthesis.

Microscopic laser surgery

Microscopic laser surgery is another innovative treatment which can be used for bulging discs in the lumbar region. Not only does it avoid the necessity for general anaesthesia, but it has the advantage of offering a more rapid recovery and reduces the likelihood of scarring.

Emergency operations for trauma and corrective surgery for medical conditions are beyond the scope of this book.

Early mobilisation following spinal surgery is essential and actively encouraged by the physiotherapists working in hospitals. In just the same way that movement and exercise should be reintroduced as soon as possible following a common-place episode of back strain, early stimulation and gentle exercise are likely to produce a far better outcome. As with recovery from any operation, the return to a pain-free existence and normal activity is better achieved with a positive approach.

Back and neck braces

Back and/or neck braces are not generally appropriate for simple back strain resulting from everyday household activities. However, I describe them here to provide an understanding of this particular treatment, should it be recommended for you, together with the type of apparatus used.

Back and neck braces are externally fitted supports, designed to restrict movement in order to help the spinal column adopt a more accurate and balanced posture. They are generally used following a traumatic injury or surgery, or to correct a spinal deformity. Records show that some form of primitive brace was used as long ago as 2000 BC.

Today, they are generally applied and fitted according to the instructions of an orthopaedic consultant, to the specific requirements of the individual patient. By restricting the position of the spine into an upright, neutral, hyper-extension (over-extended) or flexed (bent) position they can be used to achieve the corrective alignment. They are individually styled to each patient's shape and build.

There are very many different types and styles of brace. The most commonly used are listed below. Again, it is the decision of the specialist which style is most appropriate according to the diagnosis, together with the required length of time that it should be worn.

Braces might be seen as a contradictory treatment to common lower back pain where early mobility is usually recommended to aid recovery, but they have been viewed as a safe, non-invasive method of managing back pain where excessive movement might prove hazardous and risk further injury.

Although some types of brace are easily available for purchase privately, it is recommended that they should only be used following professional advice and when benefit can be closely monitored.

One exception to this is the lower-lumbar belt used by weight-lifters or those whose occupations require heavy lifting. The added support to the lower back offers increased assistance to the abdominal, thigh and back muscles in the lifting of excessive weights for the purpose of body-building and competition. These are not recommended for use therapeutically in the relief of back pain or for the prevention of its recurrence.

- **Neck braces** are generally worn to support the cervical spine. Depending on the stability of the spine, a soft collar or a halo-type brace may be used. **Halo braces** are rigid and require fixing in position by a medical professional to ensure the correct alignment of the neck vertebrae. At one time **soft collars** were recommended for use following whip-lash injuries, but this has been found to both prolong and be detrimental to the recovery of the neck tissues and gentle mobilisation is now the preferred treatment. The wearing of soft collars for other causes of neck pain or back pain is also an area of controversy since long-term benefits have not been proven.
- **Trochanteric belts**, made of thick material, are worn just below the waist and generally used to secure a fractured pelvis or to stabilise sacroiliac joints.
- **Hyper-extension braces** are another form of support for the thoracic and lumbar spine, used generally following compression fractures, or surgery where two vertebrae have been fused together. They are used to restrict forward bending and can be useful in relieving back pain.
- A similar aid is the **sacroiliac** or **lumbrosacral belt**. By putting pressure on the joints in the lumbar and sacral areas, the belt prevents excessive movement and is occasionally used to relieve lower back pain when no obvious cause can be found.
- More commonly used for low back pain are **rigid braces**. These help to keep the lumbar spine in a fixed and neutral position.

Key points

- The treatments described aim to give an understanding of some of the options available which may be prescribed to help relieve your back pain.

- Many physiotherapists specialise in musculoskeletal problems, such as back pain.

- They can provide manipulation, ultrasound and interferential (electrical current) therapy, hydrotherapy, acupuncture and active exercises to relieve pain and stiffness.

- They are highly qualified members of the medical profession.

- Tens machines give a very small electrical current through the skin in order to replace the pain signal being sent to the brain.

- Many hospitals now provide pain clinics where facet joint injections and epidurals can be given for severe back pain.

- Spinal surgery is only given after other treatments have been tried.

- There are several surgical procedures at the discretion of the surgeon, including foraminotomy, laminectomy, spine fusion, disc replacement and microscopic laser surgery.

- Back and neck braces are not generally considered suitable for nonspecific back pain.

- Braces are designed to restrict movement and in some cases their use is controversial.

Chapter 14

Complementary therapies

In the scientifically driven world that we now live in, it perhaps seems bizarre that we put faith into many of the complementary therapies that have little scientific evidence for their effectiveness. There is much written of the controversy surrounding some of the techniques, the main argument being that they work only because the recipient believes they will (known as the 'placebo effect'). For many of the lesser-known therapies, this is possibly true. It has to be remembered, however, that many of the complementary treatments have been in existence for hundreds of years and still provide both pain relief and improvement for many clients.

If you should decide to try out any of the complementary therapies described in this book, it is imperative that you are as confident as you can be that the treatment offered is both appropriate for your needs and safe. Many people decline to consult their family doctor before embarking upon a course of therapy, fearing that to suggest trying something outside the range of orthodox medicine may give rise to embarrassment or a sign of loss of confidence in other treatments. However, many experienced mainstream doctors these days are happy to support the use of some of the alternative therapies available. Indeed, there are some who may even recommend the possible benefits, if they feel it may help you.

Most doctors will have some knowledge of the methods of treatment employed and will give you important advice, especially if you have a pre-existing medical condition which might make it unwise to undertake one particular approach rather than another.

Some complementary therapies even work alongside orthodox medicine (hence the term 'complementary'), particularly chiropractic therapy and osteopathy, each of which is regulated by a professional body. Acupuncture is another alternative therapy widely acknowledged by the medical profession, but although many practitioners have been trained and belong to a reputable organisation, an overall registering body is only just being formed.

Professional therapists should be happy to provide you, as a new client, with the information you require. It is in their interest to ensure your confidence in their standard of practice.

Always ask for evidence of an individual practitioner's qualifications. Do not use any practitioner who is unqualified or fails to belong to a reputable professional body. Also, don't be afraid to ask about insurance cover for the practice – this again is for your protection in case anything goes wrong.

It is reasonable to enquire what sort of improvement can be expected following a course of treatment. This is, after all, what you are looking for. Don't spend money on an expensive course of treatment if the practitioner is uncertain whether it will help.

Cost, of course, is an important factor and may indeed influence your choice of therapy. It is clearly impossible here in this book to estimate realistically what prices may be charged for particular therapies or individual practitioners. In the United Kingdom, for example, prices range anything from £25 to £100 per session. The overall cost will also be affected by the length of each treatment and the number of return visits that may be required to achieve the desired benefits. Some therapies, however, may even be available to you through your normal health provider or insurance.

Self-help remedies and strategies may also be available, such as Tens machines, back braces and personal fitness routines from local gymnasiums. Making the right choice is therefore not so straightforward.

Since quite significant costs can be involved, it is essential that you have some understanding of the treatments available and the way in which some of the disciplines have evolved over centuries. Reflexology, for example, originated from the ancient Greeks, and Yoga from ancient India; both are more popular now than ever before. Tens machines, on the other hand, are a pain-relieving device of the 20th century.

Some treatments, particularly those involving manipulation, are not generally advised for those suffering from osteoporosis (bone thinning), severe rheumatoid arthritis (chronic inflammatory disease of joints), tumours, or osteoarthritis (joint degeneration). This is why it is so important to get a diagnosis of the cause of your back pain before embarking on treatment. However, even people who have osteoporosis are strongly advised to take some form of regular physical exercise in order to reduce the loss of minerals from their bones. This not only improves strength and muscle tone, but helps to maintain good balance, which, in the elderly, can prevent susceptibility to falls.

Personal knowledge from family members and friends is a very useful resource. There is nothing like the passing on of individual experience to help in your decision-making, though at the same time you should not forget that individual cases are purely illustrative and cannot prove that any particular treatment will be appropriate in your case.

I do not make any recommendations in this section of the book; I purely set out to give a brief outline of the various techniques and programmes most widely available, together with their historical origins. Sources of further information are included in the Appendix for readers who want to find out more about any particular approach. There are very many more complementary therapies besides those included here, but to describe them all would only add to the confusion. Therefore I have described only those therapies that are administered by qualified practitioners and are mostly registered by a governing body. They are set out in alphabetical order.

Acupuncture

History

The very word 'acupuncture' used to conjure up suspicion and apprehension, but this is now one of the most well-respected forms of complementary therapy. Discovered in China over 3000 years ago, it was brought to Europe by Chinese practitioners in the 19th century. It did not, however, become popular until President Nixon's visit to China in 1972.

Acupuncture has now seen the development of clinics throughout the world and its benefits are widely acknowledged. In the past two decades it has begun to feature more prominently in mainstream healthcare in the UK. The World Health Organisation supports its use and it unites both mainstream and alternative healthcare practitioners. Increasingly, health professionals, such as doctors, nurses, midwives and dentists, use or recommend it as an effective treatment for pain and other health problems.

Principles, mode of action and evidence

An increasing weight of evidence from Western scientific research is demonstrating the effectiveness of acupuncture for treating a wide variety of conditions (e.g. Linde et al, 2009), of which back pain is just one. Further trials are still needed, but several positive results seem to demonstrate that it provides more than the placebo effect (as explained above) (Furlan et al, 2010). In the UK, the National Institute for Health and Clinical Excellence recently recommended 10 weekly sessions of acupuncture over a period of 12 weeks as a first line treatment modality for non-specific low back pain (NICE 2009). A course of treatment may be offered to you by your healthcare team if low back pain has been present for more than six weeks.

From a biomedical viewpoint, it is believed to stimulate the nervous system, influencing the production of the body's communication substances – hormones and neurotransmitters. The resulting biochemical changes activate the body's self-regulating homeostatic (balancing) systems, stimulating its natural healing abilities and promoting physical and emotional wellbeing.

What the treatment involves

Commonly used in the treatment of back pain, fine needles are inserted into specific points in the body, where they are left in place for anything from 10 to 30 minutes.

Acupuncture needles average 4 to 5 centimetres in length, are very thin, almost hair-like, made mostly of stainless steel, and should always be 'single use' only. Sessions typically last from 20 to 30 minutes, and a course of up to 10 sessions is usual.

Some acupuncturists ask for a medical questionnaire to be completed prior to an initial appointment, whilst others allow time for a detailed interview to both correctly diagnose your problem and to identify any risk factors which may make acupuncture inappropriate.

Training for practitioners

Qualifications for acupuncturists vary. In the UK, qualified medical professionals usually undertake training through the British Medical Acupuncture Society, whilst others train in traditional Chinese acupuncture through the British Acupuncture Council. Medical acupuncture, which evolved from traditional Chinese acupuncture, is the form that is practised predominantly by conventionally trained healthcare practitioners in Western countries, using current knowledge of anatomy, physiology and pathology and the principles of evidence-based medicine.

Licensing still varies from country to country, but with the introduction of a professional registering body (British Acupuncture Council), although some practitioners are registered with the Association of Traditional Chinese Medicine, it is anticipated that soon there will be uniformity within the practice. This will help eliminate those who describe themselves as acupuncturists but hold no certification of competence.

Potential risks

Unlike other complementary therapies, as acupuncture involves a form of invasive procedure (pricking the skin with needles), it is of greater importance that the environment where the treatment is carried out is suitable. In order to reduce the risk of cross-infection, the room should be as you would expect of any clinical treatment room. That is to say, with a clean, washable floor, basin for hand washing, and adequate lighting. The needles should be produced from new, sealed packs and disposed of into a suitable 'sharps' container after use.

It should be remembered that, as with other types of pain relief, relieving the symptoms is only half the battle. Improved posture and appropriate exercises are also necessary in order to strengthen the body and help prevent the return of the pain.

Alexander technique

History

The Alexander technique is a method of recognising habitual tensions and relieving them through coordinated breathing, posture and movement. Practitioners claim the therapeutic effects of eased breathing and movement, and reduced back pain.

The technique is named after Frederick Matthias Alexander (1869–1955), who developed it initially as a personal tool to alleviate his own breathing problems and voice-hoarseness in order to help his passion for Shakespearean acting. Alexander believed his work could be applied to improve individual health and wellbeing, and further refined his approach of self-observation and re-training for wider use. He developed his technique in Australia but in 1904 came to London where he continued to practise until his death in 1955. He published his experiences in four books, *Man's Supreme Inheritance* (1910), *Addendum* (1911), *Conscious Control* (1912), and a combined volume in 1918. He also trained individuals to teach the technique.

Principles, mode of action and evidence

The Alexander technique is used remedially to regain freedom of movement. It is used to undo the establishment of nuisance habits and to develop self-awareness; it can provide a self-help tool to change specific habits. These elements may help in alleviating pain and weakness as a result of poor posture or repetitive physical demands, and can improve pain management in chronic disability. The Alexander technique has been shown to be an effective treatment for chronic or recurrent back pain in a recent randomised study (Little P, 2008).

What the treatment involves

In most cases, individuals must pay for their Alexander technique education. Those who are used to getting instant results may complain at having to commit to 20–40 private (one-to-one) lessons, which is the duration most Alexander teachers recommend is required to gain proficiency. Workshops do exist, but usually do not last long enough to fulfil most students' educational requirements; they will need to attend additional private lessons if they want to gain proficiency.

Training for practitioners

The London Centre for Alexander Technique and Training offers courses of 1600 hours over a period of three years, from which students gain membership to the Society of Teachers of the Alexander Technique.

Potential risks

There are no reports of effects detrimental to health relating to the Alexander technique. Since there is no invasive or forceful treatment involved, but techniques involving breathing, vocal and tension patterns, and movement, it would appear to be a safe and gentle method.

Chiropractic therapy

History

Of all the many and varied complementary medicines, chiropractic therapy is one of the most widely known and practised in the West. These days many orthodox doctors recommend it as a beneficial treatment for painful necks and backs.

Chiropractic therapy was founded in 1865 in the USA by a Canadian called Daniel P Palmer. Palmer (a man of dubious character), worked for a time as a magnetic healer. He developed the theory that manipulation of the spine was effective in healing many ailments, even including deafness and heart conditions. He believed that most human ailments were derived from friction of the nerves caused by the displacement of vertebrae, which in turn led to inflammation and disease affecting internal organ function. His introduction of the word 'subluxation' was used to describe the way misaligned spinal vertebrae could interfere with their surrounding nerves. Palmer, whose early therapy was seen as 'practising medicine without a proper licence', opened colleges in which to educate others in his techniques, incorporating some of the ideas from naturopathy and osteopathy into his treatments.

Palmer's original concept of chiropractic treatment was developed based on the idea that if spinal or other joint misalignment was corrected, normal nerve function, inflammation and pain would be relieved as a result. Whilst this basic hypothesis is still the underlying philosophy, much of Palmer's original ideas regarding how chiropractic therapy worked have now been discarded as more scientific reasoning has improved understanding of the physiological mechanisms of pain and its control.

Principles, mode of action and evidence

The aim of the treatment, after identifying areas of muscle tension and pain, is to relax the muscles and free any locked joints by gentle manipulation, generally carried out in a series of sessions over a period of several weeks. (It should of course be noted that while it aims to tackle muscle spasm and inflammation, and thereby relieve pain, it does not set out to strengthen muscles or change habits that are risky for future episodes of back pain.)

Both chiropractors and osteopaths use manual palpation to identify areas of sensitivity or inflammation. This method of diagnosis also establishes details relating to the structural alignment of the bones. Clients are usually asked to walk, bend and move their spine in various directions in order to demonstrate the limits of their mobility so that the full extent of the problem can be ascertained before treatment commences.

Chiropractic manipulation aims to open up the spaces between the spinal vertebrae, or loosen stiff joints, in order to improve flexibility and restore normal function. These techniques also aim to change the nerve messages being sent from the spine to the brain by stimulating the joint movement receptors, which can affect nerve irritation and help relieve pain.

These days the greater proportion of a chiropractor's work is for the treatment of back and neck pain. Studies carried out in Australia, UK and USA have shown very positive benefits in the treatment of low back pain but, as with many other complementary therapies, negative studies also exist stating that such evidence is inconclusive and weak. The British Chiropractic Association Research quotes a considerable number of positive reviews, including the NICE Guidelines 2009, and the UK BEAM trial 2004 (www.chiropractic-uk.co.uk/Research). However, Jha A (2007), *Guardian*, disputes the evidence that chiropractic is helpful for back pain.

Training for practitioners

It was not until the early 1900s that chiropractic therapy was introduced to the United Kingdom. The British Chiropractic Association was subsequently formed in 1925 to regulate standards of practice. In 1994, a UK Act of Parliament was introduced to ensure that all chiropractors should be registered, following an intense period of training. Today, training to be a chiropractor involves a four- or five-year degree course, which also includes some traditional clinical training.

What the treatment involves

Private chiropractic clinics are widely available in many countries, and demand for their services is increasing all the time. Although not cheap, the epidemic rise in the number of people with back pain makes this method of spinal realignment and its subsequent relief of acute pain ever more popular. Chiropractic sessions generally take approximately 15–20 minutes, although an initial visit can take up to an hour to allow for a full medical history and physical examination to determine a correct diagnosis and discuss with the recipient appropriate treatment.

Potential risks

Despite the many reports of benefits and improved health resulting from chiropractic therapy, there still remains a question mark over its safety. Articles written by Rubinstein SM (2008) and by Ernst E (2007) and (2010) still challenge the occurrence of adverse effects of spinal manipulation and that of cerebral vascular accidents (strokes) following manipulation of the neck.

Manipulation, by its very nature, is a procedure likely to be uncomfortable when it is carried out, but the overall opinion of research would suggest that the treatment itself is beneficial in most cases.

Hypnotherapy

History

Hypnosis is another modality that can be a useful means of treating acute pain and beneficial in lowering the need for medications. It is also a means of providing relaxation to tense muscles and can aid more restful sleep.

It is unclear exactly when the ability to hypnotise another person was first recognised. Certainly it would appear to have been in existence, in one form or another, for very many centuries, and throughout the world. 'Hypno' comes from Ancient Greek, meaning 'to sleep', but records have shown evidence of 'trance-like' states being induced over the centuries in individuals in places as diverse as Australia, Africa, India and Egypt.

Dr Franz Anton Mesmer, of Swiss-German origin and from whom the term 'mesmerise' was derived, is perhaps the most renowned initiator of the practice as we know it today. He practised in Vienna in the 18th century and was particularly interested in 'magnetic medicine' which involved passing magnets over the body to effect healing. Many others, however, are credited with influencing the development of hypnotherapy, including the Scot, James Braid, and James Esdaile in India, who were among the first to bring a more scientific approach to hypnosis.

Principles, mode of action and evidence

Today, hypnotherapy is occasionally used in dentistry or for those suffering phobias or extreme anxiety. It is said that by reducing anxiety according to the principles described below, it also reduces the significance of pain to the individual. Whilst perhaps not eliminating the pain altogether, the aim is to return control of it back to the sufferer, instead of allowing the pain to be the dominant factor limiting mobility.

Hypnosis works by creating a mental state in which the subconscious mind is opened to the power of suggestion during a state of deep relaxation. In this way, the mind can be influenced to respond to the pain messages by programming the brain to release endorphins that will relieve the discomfort. Endorphins are the body's own naturally produced pain-blocking substance and act in a similar way to opiate-like drugs, such as morphine. The release of endorphins in the body is often said to give rise to a sense of euphoria in athletes, who can suffer great discomfort during extreme physical training.

Several clinical trials have been undertaken, mostly showing that hypnosis significantly reduces pain and can be more effective than other treatments, such as physiotherapy. However, there is a lack of standardisation of the hypnotic interventions which have been examined in the clinical trials, making the results confusing. This is often due to the fact that sufferers of chronic pain are taught to carry out self-hypnosis as part of their treatment, which makes accurate analysis difficult (www.ncbi.nim.nih.gov/pubmed 20183738).

What the treatment involves

Hypnosis is usually carried out while the recipient is in a fully conscious state. Some people, however, enter a deep trance and have no recollection of what has been said or done. Studies (www.hypnosis.me.uk.pages/research.html) have shown that whilst in such a state, there is a change in brain chemistry and brain waves which cause the release of endorphins and it is suggested that this is responsible for achieving complete relaxation.

Typically, a hypnotherapy session lasts at least 45 minutes, sometimes over an hour, and like other private therapies the number of sessions can vary until the optimum benefit is perceived to have been achieved. These sessions are usually provided in the premises of the hypnotist, but can sometimes be carried out in the client's own home. Charges vary considerably, which may relate to the experience, success rate and/or training of the individual therapist.

Training for practitioners

Unlike other specialist complementary therapies, there is no legal requirement for a hypnotist to be qualified, and care should be taken in selecting a suitable therapist. Personal recommendation from a friend or family member is probably a very valuable guide, although there are many therapists who have undergone an approved course of training. The National Council for Hypnotherapy offers courses through accredited training schools, which in turn offer 120–450 study hours towards the independently verified 'Hypnotherapy Practitioner Diploma'. Although there is no regulation of the profession, there are national occupational standards to protect both clients and practitioners.

Potential risks

Hypnotherapy holds many anxieties for some (usually fear of saying or doing something silly) but this technique is not for entertainment or fun; it is purely to relieve pain. There is no guarantee that it is always successful, but if it reduces the amount of analgesic medication required to manage your pain and gives sufficient relief for you to tolerate exercise and mobility, then maybe it is worth a try.

However, there are risks attached to using hypnotherapy as a treatment for back pain. Despite claims made for its effectiveness, sometimes even as a complete cure, it is unsafe to eliminate the pain without first addressing its cause. Pain is a symptom that something is wrong. If the pain is removed, it is possible to mask an underlying cause that may need conventional medical treatment or even surgery or chemotherapy.

(At the same time, there is also evidence that pain can sometimes be a problem just of the brain. In this situation, even if there is no physical cause found, the brain may continue to experience the pain and, left untreated, this can become chronic or even permanent.)

Massage

History

There are many different forms of massage, some of which have been incorporated into the treatments of chiropractic and osteopathy. It is, however, a complementary therapy in its own right.

The word massage is thought to be derived from either the Greek word 'masso' meaning 'to knead' or the Arabic 'mas'h' which means 'to touch, feel or handle'. Evidence of massage, found in both China and Egypt, describes its use as far back as 400 BC, and there are hints of this type of therapy that can be traced back as far as 2,500 BC.

Throughout the centuries, many different types of massage have been developed. Each type pertains to a different part of the world, including Japan, where Shiatsu, a form of finger or acupressure, was practised; China, which incorporated a variety of methods of massage and relaxation; and India, where practitioners focused on Ayurvedic, a more sensual massage approach. In the West, where this practice has most recently been adopted, practitioners use effleurage (stroking), squeezing and striking (see below). Today massage is not only used to relax muscles and relieve pain, including back pain, arthritis and inflammation, but it has also become popularised in beauty salons, sports centres and many other community facilities.

Principles, mode of action and evidence

Massage works by stimulating the body's own natural pain killers, known as endorphins, providing a 'feel good' sensation. This calm and relaxing motion, with its smooth and rhythmic waves of pressure, has many benefits apart from the release of muscular tension and pain. The increased circulation to the area brings with it a boost of nutrients to the damaged tissues. It is also said to reduce anxiety and aid more restful sleep.

What the treatment involves

With nearly 30 different types of massage to choose from, the techniques are similarly diverse. (See below for the most relevant to back pain.) They differ in the amount of pressure and stretching movements, known as the 'mechanical action', and in the body's own response to the stimulation of the nerve receptors, known as the 'reflex action'. Techniques range from gentle massage strokes to more vigorous kneading, rubbing or tapping actions, depending on the condition to be treated. Reflexology and finger pressure applied to pressure points (known as meridians) also demonstrate a close association with other complementary therapies.

One of the most popular therapeutic massages used today was that developed at the end of the 19th century by a Swedish physical educator, Per Henrik Ling, who is also documented as founding physical therapy (see 'physiotherapy', page 103). Ling's method encompasses five basic elements: 'Effleurage', which is gentle stroking to relax muscles; 'Petrissage', which is the kneading and squeezing of soft tissue; 'Friction and Compression', which entails rubbing and holding; 'Tapotement', which describes tapping movements using the side of the hand or heel of the palm; and 'Vibration', which involves using rapid rhythmical movements to release tension.

The type of massage to be used depends on both the diagnosis and the preferred method of the therapist. For some techniques it is necessary to be unclothed, although towels will be used to protect your dignity. In this case, massage oils are applied to the hands of the therapist to allow the muscles to be manipulated from gentle strokes to more vigorous kneading in a constant movement. For other techniques, loose cotton clothing is acceptable. If you are uncomfortable with this aspect of the therapy it is wise to consult your practitioner before embarking on this type of treatment.

The relevant options for back pain resulting from back strain include the following:

• **Remedial massage** aims specifically to work on joints and muscles which have suffered injury. By massaging stiff and painful tissue, there is an increase in blood and lymph circulation to the area. This in turn aids the removal of waste products which may also help reduce excess fluids causing swelling.

• **Ice massage** is the application of an ice pack to that part of the back where the pain is more severe. A cold compress given in this way helps to reduce inflammation following recent injury. Although the circulation contracts away from the area due to contact with the cold pack, when it is removed the returning rush of blood to the area brings with it an increase of nutrients to the area. The great advantage to this treatment is that it can be self-administered at home and is free. Care must be taken, however, not to place the ice pack directly onto the skin as it can burn. Wrap it in a towel or other suitable material. Frequent, short applications of no more than 10 minutes of the ice pack are preferable, rather than a prolonged session. Ice packs should not be used if there are any symptoms of numbness, altered sensation to the area following the injury or medical conditions, such as Raynaud's disease or arthritis.

• **Massage chairs** are a more recent method of massage therapy which involves the use of electrically controlled vibration. For some sufferers of back pain they can provide good relief. This alternative type of massage treatment is sometimes available for use in private clinics, but they are also available for purchase and use in the privacy of your home. They are expensive, however, and you are well advised to try one out to see whether sufficient relief is gained before laying out such expense, as they do not help everyone. Also, massage chairs should not be purchased without first gaining medical advice, since there are some health circumstances which render this treatment unsuitable. These include the aftermath of chemotherapy, radiation or recent fracture. If you do decide to go ahead with buying your own, ensure that adequate training in the correct use of the chair is provided by the supplier as well as appropriate future servicing requirements.

Training and accreditation of practitioners

A word of caution: although most massage therapists in the United Kingdom are listed on a national register, are bound by a code of conduct and have completed training at an approved establishment, this is not compulsory. This means that without the existence of a single regulatory body, anybody can set up as a massage therapist. In the UK, there are several associations for massage therapists. These include the General Council for Massage Therapies, the National Association of Massage & Manipulative Therapists, and Massage Therapy UK. Several organisations also exist in Australia, Canada, the United States and New Zealand. It is advisable to check out the credentials of your local practitioner, to ascertain his/her qualifications and experience, and whether he/she holds indemnity insurance, as well as the costs involved beforehand.

With this in mind, self-help books are available (see Appendix for some suggestions). Such books fully explain some of the simpler techniques which require the assistance of one helper and the recipient. Some methods of self-massage are also available in this way, which may provide some relief from pain.

Osteopathy

History

Osteopathy is a therapy based on manipulation of bones and joints, including the treatment of muscles, ligaments and connective tissues. Very similar to chiropractic therapy, its purpose is to correct misalignment of bones and treat the problems associated with injury, in order to return normal function and allow healing. The word 'osteopathy' is derived from the Ancient Greek words 'osteon' meaning 'bone' and 'pathos' meaning 'disease or suffering'.

Just like chiropractic therapy, osteopathy was founded in the United States of America. Its conception in 1890 was by Dr Andrew Still, from Missouri, who sought a new method of treatment for the skeletal and nervous system. Disillusioned with current medical techniques at that time, and following the deaths of his wife and three of his own children, he worked on the principle that the body was able to heal itself provided it was structurally sound and balanced.

As with chiropractic therapy, he considered that all disease could be related to a structural imbalance within the human frame, which in turn affected the nerve and blood supply to the major organs of the body. He called these imbalances 'osteopathic lesions'. In order to increase mobility, relieve tension and blockages, as well as improve the flow of blood and lymph, he formulated a system of manipulation, stretching and massages. His original philosophy is still fundamental to modern-day osteopathy, but has developed to incorporate many new techniques and approaches.

Principles, mode of action and evidence

The aim of a manipulation is to release muscular tension or spasm in order to restore mobility and improve circulation. One technique, called 'high velocity low amplitude thrust', involves applying a rapid thrust to a joint or misaligned spinal bone. Although not particularly painful, a crack or popping sound can sometimes be heard as the tissues are released. For some recipients, relief and increased flexibility are said to be immediate.

You might be forgiven for thinking that osteopathy and chiropractic are very similar in their holistic methods of treatment, since both complementary therapies are also concerned with diet, lifestyle and the emotional wellbeing of clients. Indeed, some osteopathic techniques have been incorporated into chiropractic therapy. As a rudimentary guide to their differences, an osteopath manipulates using leverage close to a joint, whereas a chiropractor manipulates directly over a joint. Apart from manipulation, osteopaths use other techniques such as stretching, pressure and mobilisation. Another difference is that osteopaths do not 'click back' a joint the way chiropractors do.

Treatment for acute back pain is, perhaps, the best known therapy provided by osteopaths, but increasingly more and more people are attending osteopathy clinics for all kinds of medical problems, ranging from whiplash and joint injuries to digestive problems, asthma and many others.

As with other complementary therapies, its close association with conventional medicine has been accepted now for many years, with many physicians also learning the skills of osteopathy. Occasionally research trials have brought into question the efficacy and cost of osteopathy (Licciardone JC (2007), Williams NH (2004)), but generally its reputation has remained unscathed.

What the treatment involves

An initial consultation with an osteopath can be lengthy. A thorough and detailed medical history, visual observations of posture and movement, assessment of blood pressure and possibly X-rays, determine the diagnosis on the basis of which appropriate treatment is planned. Depending upon the problem identified, one of several techniques may be initiated.

- **Relaxation** – Kneading actions, stretching and rolling in a manner ranging from mild to more vigorous movements are used to relax soft tissue and muscles.
- Loosening tight joints can be effected by mobilising the joint through its full range of movement. This action is called **'articulation'** and benefits the muscles and ligaments too.
- **Manipulation** is perhaps the technique for which osteopathy is most renowned. This entails a sudden thrust which is given to return a displaced joint to its correct position. This can sometimes be momentarily uncomfortable, but more gentle manipulative leverage is also sometimes employed.
- Other treatments include massage, direct pressure to certain trigger points and the manual contraction and stretching of tense muscles.
- **'Myofascial' release** is a method of stretching and easing out of muscles which also releases tension and increases the range of movement.

Such treatment sessions can take from 20 to 60 minutes, depending on the problem diagnosed, which will also dictate the number of follow-up sessions required. Clinics local to your area can be found listed in telephone directories or may even be recommended by a doctor. Many leisure and sports clubs also have osteopaths linked to their organisations who will often accept outside clients requiring treatment.

Osteopathic treatment can be quite expensive. Although the number of sessions required will depend on the individual's requirements, typically three to six sessions over a period of six to eight weeks is average.

Training for practitioners

As with other therapeutic treatments, such as physiotherapy and chiropractic therapy, a lengthy degree level course is required for qualification. The letters displayed after the practitioner's names may be seen to differ. DO (Diploma of Osteopathy), BSc Ost (Batchelor of Science specialising in osteopathy) are most usual in the UK, and others exist where training was acquired in other countries – for example, DAAO or DOM in Germany and OCNZ in New Zealand. This is sometimes because different educational establishments have awarded individually recognised qualifications. It may also reflect the length of time since the qualification was gained. Nevertheless, all appropriately trained practitioners are registered with their professional body of osteopaths, which in the UK is the General Osteopathic Council.

Potential risks

There is a small element of risk. Generally only minor side effects, such as bruising, tiredness or headache, are likely, but rarely, complications such as damage to an artery, a stroke or compression of the nerves at the base of the spinal cord have been reported (www.bupa.co.uk). For this reason it is imperative that a full examination is carried out prior to treatment and existing medical conditions are taken into consideration.

Pilates

History

One of the most successful and popular methods of exercise to both prevent and alleviate back problems is Pilates. Throughout many countries, in towns and villages, specially trained Pilates teachers run courses in gymnasiums, village halls, schools and other community-based venues for anyone concerned about back problems. Several self-help books have also been produced (see Appendix).

It is a fairly recent discipline, and conceived as the result of the fascinating personal experiences of Joseph Pilates, who originated from Dusseldorf in Germany. As a frail and weak youngster, he initially took up body-building to improve his own strength and developed to become good all-round sportsman. After moving to England in 1912, the outbreak of the First World War meant that as a German, he was interned and used this period of time to further develop his techniques for achieving physical fitness. Later, working as a nurse, in his efforts to rehabilitate injured soldiers returning from the conflict, he began by using a system of strings and pulleys that could be used by bed-ridden victims in order to maintain muscle tone without risking further injury. He initially called his methods 'muscle contrology'.

In New York, after the war, his techniques proved successful with many professional dancers and when its benefits were discovered by sportsmen and others, he saw his approach to holistic fitness grow in popularity across all society. The popularity of his methods has continued to grow and his successors have continued to refine his original philosophy, pursuing his endeavour to help individuals overcome their physical limitations.

Joseph Pilates also discovered in his early method of exercise that springs were useful as a means of creating resistance. He found they could be used to encourage muscle control to be exercised both with and against the equipment. In this way, personal benefit was achieved by exerting energy to use the spring, thus making the body work the apparatus, rather than depending upon the apparatus to work for the body.

Unlike his earlier efforts, the exercises of today do not require fancy or cumbersome equipment. Some exercise programmes, however, can include the use of a stretch band or an inflatable ball. It is the use of stretch bands, which can be employed to strengthen and tone the body, that simulates Pilates' original use of springs to provide resistance against movement. Similarly, it is the individual's pressure applied to an inflatable ball, rather than the ball itself, that provides a means of exercise.

All that is basically necessary is an exercise mat and comfortable loose clothing. A series of choreographed movements, appropriate to the limitations of the individual, can increase in intensity or difficulty as the recipient's fitness improves.

Principles, mode of action and evidence

Pilates exercises work on improving the **'girdle of strength'**. This term relates to the three main areas responsible for posture, strength and flexibility – namely, the abdomen, back and buttocks. It is fair to say that most beneficial exercises designed to prevent or recover from back pain are similar to or based upon the tested theories of this practice. Great emphasis is put on the correction of posture, with a strong but relaxed alignment of the spine, together with the importance of maintaining this attitude during normal daily life. Its benefits as a fitness regime are also well documented (www.nhs./livewell/fitness/pilates.aspx).

Five main principles underpin the Pilates method.

• **First principle: concentration** – The importance of concentration is stressed since awareness of your own body in making certain that every part of it is moved or positioned correctly not only ensures that each element of the exercises is accurately maintained, but promotes relief from other concerns or anxieties in life that may be giving rise to tension.

• **Second principle: effective breathing** – Effective breathing is another technique taught. Contrary to the short superficial breaths most of us take naturally, Pilates exercises encourage deep rhythmic breathing, using the full capacity of the lungs and with the emphasis on using the effort to breathe out rather than in. Movement is always carried out on an outward breath. In this way, it is possible to avoid any tension created by taking a breath in at the same time as the effort of the exercise.

• **Third principle: the 'girdle of strength'** – Pilates' emphasis on the 'girdle of strength' is fundamental to every movement by always combining the involvement of the back, abdomen and buttocks. Nearly every exercise of Pilates begins by drawing the navel gently in towards the spine, which, as demonstrated earlier in the book, engages the abdominal muscles to protect and strengthen the back. By also clenching the buttock muscles it creates an extremely strong foundation for almost any exercise.

• **Fourth principle: flowing movements** – The aim is to achieve flowing movements by letting one exercise position flow slowly and naturally into the next in time with your own breathing. This avoids any sudden changes. In this way, the precision of the exercises is kept co-ordinated and smooth.

• **Fifth principle: relaxation** – Lastly, relaxation and breathing exercises are an essential part of Pilates. The relief of mental stress, tense muscles and pain from injury, forms the basis of this very popular and successful method.

What the treatment involves

Pilates exercises are designed to relieve tension throughout the body, but particularly in the back, shoulders and neck by using a slow and relaxing rhythm. Stiff joints and frozen muscles can be very successfully treated by adopting the methods taught in Pilates and as such it is a very popular form of regular exercise.

It is not an aerobic form of exercise, nor does it over-develop some parts of the body whilst neglecting others. Whilst focusing on core strength, it promotes muscle development, flexibility and improved mobility of all the joints. For this reason many athletes find this method of exercise particularly helpful.

The principles of Pilates' exercises have changed little over the years, still offering a method of gentle and supportive exercise appropriate for all ages and levels of general fitness. Although a modest cost is involved, it is always recommended that an initial course, run by a trained instructor, should be undertaken before embarking on the use of self-help books and videos (see Appendix). It is imperative that correct alignment and posture are learnt under the guidance of an expert before trying other exercises and stretch movements. It is also acknowledged that as a regular and a social activity, the impetus to work at strengthening the core muscles and improve posture are more likely to be maintained in a group and in the presence of an instructor, rather than when simply trying to imitate pictures of such exacting positions in a book with the aid of a mirror. However, many books and videos (see Appendix) offer excellent guidance and advice for continued improvement. Mixed-level classes for all ages and abilities are common, but many teachers also provide sessions for small groups of beginners and for those whose lifestyles restrict their access to classes.

Training for practioners

There would appear to be a vast range in the competencies required for Pilates teachers. Training can vary from a university four-year degree course, to studying from home over a period of a few weeks. There are several establishments in the UK who offer regulated training for Pilates instructors and are bound by a code of ethics and conduct. These trainers will be registered with the Pilates Foundation, London.

Potential risks

Again, as with other complementary therapies, there are research reports which claim that Pilates is not beneficial, indeed some would go so far as to say it is detrimental to your back (Graves S (2005), www.dailymail.co.uk/article 440309/1s (2007)). Therefore your Pilates instructor must be made aware of any previous or existing back problems that you may have before commencing any programme of exercise.

Reflexology

History

Reflexology is the practice of influencing health by applying pressure to specific points on the hands and feet which are considered to correspond to different parts of the body via nerve pathways. Popularised in the West in the 1930s, we know it as a fairly modern concept, but its true origins can be traced back as far as the Egyptians in 2330 BC and the Ancient Chinese, some 5000 years ago. Evidence too has been found in Japan and other eastern countries, where stone and etched footprints signified the custom of walking barefoot on natural surfaces as a means of benefiting the health of the body.

Mode of action and evidence

Many Western medical practitioners and scientists have more recently developed the theory that direct pressure applied to parts of the foot or hand can lessen the pain in its corresponding area. An intricate map of the external surfaces of both hands and feet illustrate a complex chart of irregularly shaped and sized areas, each denoting the various reflex zones and their corresponding parts of the body. Pressure areas identified on the right hand or foot correlate to the appropriate region or organ on the right side of the body.

The technique used aims to stimulate the nerves, which travel to the parts of the brain that are thought to be responsible for tension in specific zones of the body, by using the flow of energy through the body along channels, also known as 'meridians' or 'health pathways'.

Over the past decades, many international studies (www.reflexology-research.com/whatis.htm) have shown very positive results from this 'healing hands' approach, but there still exists considerable scepticism amongst many in the medical profession, who express concern that, whilst reflexology can do no harm, its place as a recognised method of successful treatment has still to be proved (Ernst E (2009)). Without significant evidence of its benefits, there is a worry that serious illnesses may go undiagnosed and untreated without the benefit of modern medical science.

What the treatment involves

There are many reasons why people, from all walks of life, turn to reflexology. It is popular for its natural, drug-free and non-intrusive approach to maintaining good health and relaxation. It is also used by many who pursue its potential healing powers when more orthodox methods of treatment appear to have failed or given little relief. Without doubt it offers an enormously increased feeling of relaxation, releasing stress and tension for many. In the past few years the technique has become an extremely valuable addition to the care and treatment afforded to patients with chronic or terminal illnesses. The added ability of a friend or relative to participate in administering this care has been regularly demonstrated to reduce pain and improve emotional contentment. In the early stages of back pain, when muscle spasm is at its worst, this supplementary treatment can only be beneficial.

Unlike some other therapies, such as Yoga or Pilates, this is a treatment generally carried out on a one-to-one basis in a clinical setting between the recipient and a trained practitioner. Sessions normally take about 30 to 45 minutes and you should begin to feel its benefits within two or three visits. Charges vary significantly from one clinic to another and it is recommended that questions relating to cost as well as the training (see below) and length of experience of the practitioner should be explored prior to booking.

Training for practitioners

The length of training for a reflexologist is varied. In some cases, a weekend course has been considered sufficient to qualify someone to practise, whereas others have completed 50 hours' instruction or more intense training. In some situations, a concerned friend or relative is able to participate alongside the professional reflexologist, emulating and supporting the therapy. Such an additional contribution may not only help to improve a patient's quality of life, but can provide a positive and emotionally supportive role for the carer. Self-help methods can also be taught and there are many books available (see the Appendix for some suggestions) which provide clear and illustrated instruction.

Potential risks

Due to the lack of regulated medical training for many reflexologists, it is not surprising that the main concern amongst physicians is that whilst reflexology therapy is not likely to cause harm, it is possible that it may cause a delay in the diagnosis of a serious medical condition.

Yoga

History

The complementary therapy of Yoga originated in India and is thought to have been practised as long ago as 3000 BC to promote physical and spiritual health. The word 'yoga' comes from a Sanskrit word meaning 'union', signifying the union of body, mind and spirit. The first known text was written about 200 BC by a legendary yogi called Patanjali, who described the principles of physical and spiritual health using the methods called Yoga Sutras.

Yoga did not reach the West until about the 1960s but was quickly popularised by celebrities and rock stars who saw it as a somewhat exotic alternative lifestyle to that of materialistic stardom. Today, Yoga is a popular and widely respected form of physical exercise which encompasses relaxation, meditation, diet, massage and breathing control.

Principles and mode of action

Yoga claims to be a powerful, holistic and transforming tool which concentrates on its therapeutic benefits, offering a treatment programme to treat aches, pains and fatigue. The aim is to improve your general health as well as the problem. In order that all the muscle groups of the body are stimulated equally, rather than encouraging the overworking of some muscle groups whilst neglecting others, the programme is designed to incorporate the whole body.

There are many different types of Yoga. **Hatha Yoga** is one of the most popular used in the West. Developed in the 15th century in India, it is based upon employing a series of body poses called 'asanas'. They range from simple positions to more advanced postures, which are either held statically or performed in an active sequence. It is claimed that the practice of Yoga asanas can have the effect of slowing brain waves, heart beat and respiration rate which, together with reduced muscle tension and stress, creates both an overall improvement in health and a sense of wellbeing.

Yoga carries the belief that we all have a healing force or 'sanogenetic power' within us. Aspects of our lives that cause damage to our health, like stress, bacteria, lack of sleep and an excessive intake of alcohol, are believed to fight against this innate power. Yoga aims to create a feeling of wellbeing which is capable of preventing and curing illness by encouraging the body to feel good and energetic. **Therapeutic Yoga** focuses on specific illnesses, both chronic and acute, and aims to cure them with a tailor-made exercise programme.

The effects of Yoga on the body are described as direct, indirect and a combination of the two. As a **direct effect**, stretching and strengthening exercises are used to alleviate the pain and stiffness of back pain, as well as developing the muscles to prevent a recurrence. The **indirect effect** goes further, using numerous Yoga postures to improve blood flow to the brain. Yogic breathing exercises are used to reduce anxiety, producing a beneficial calming effect both physically and spiritually.

It is the **combination** of these two effects that is used to prevent and combat many illnesses and physical conditions. The purpose is to gently increase breath control to improve the health and function of both body and mind. These two systems of exercise and breathing then prepare the body and mind for meditation (www.amercanyogaassociation.org/general.html).

What the practice of Yoga involves

Yogic principles include a vegetarian diet and recommend fasting one day a week. This does not mean the exclusion of all foods, but restricting oneself to consuming only non-citric fruits, green salads, vegetable soups and herbal teas. These dietary requirements, together with meditation, are also used as a preventative measure to lower high blood pressure, since the relieving of stress within the body is essential in the prevention of many ailments, including back pain.

Much credence is also given to the benefits of therapeutic massage, either by a general massage provided by a helper, or self-massage. Self-massage can also be taught as an effective treatment of a specific area of the body in order to stimulate healing by improving blood circulation to that region.

Modestly priced classes are available in most towns and cities across the world and self-help books and videos (see Appendix) are also available for those who prefer to copy and practise the exercises and advice at home. Just like Pilates, however, trained personnel are the ideal instructors for the novice, as it is imperative that correct posture and advice are followed. Courses give added support and encouragement, where questions can be answered, as well as the opportunity to make new friendships with others making similar lifestyle changes.

Training for practitioners/instructors

The training of Yoga teachers is varied and carried out in very many organisations. The most widely recognised qualification in the UK is the British Wheel of Yoga, which is currently undergoing international affiliation. This accredited school awards successful graduates, following 200 hours of training, the entitlement to display RYT. They are covered by UK teaching insurance and can display the Yoga Alliance logo.

Potential risks

Risks associated with Yoga are ignorance of pre-existing health conditions, and an inappropriate level of fitness and stretching past our normal limits, causing strain. This is corroborated by the American Academy of Orthopaedic Surgeons, who quote common injuries to neck, shoulders and spine. (www.care2.com/ avoiding-the-dangers-of-yoga).

Other complementary therapies

There are many less well-known complementary therapies, each with varying approaches to combating the problems of back strain. A very brief description of some of these is shown below.

• The **Feldenkrais** technique was inspired by a Ukrainian, Moshe´ Feldenkrais (1904-1984), who was a physicist, engineer and judo master. In the 1940s, his method of 'awareness through movement' became an increasingly popular method of treating back pain and tension. The treatment, which consists mainly of gentle manipulation and exercises, is said to restore mobility by correcting imbalance within the nervous system.

- A similar technique, called the **Hellerwork**, also involves manipulation to realign the body and release muscle tension. Deep pressure is also applied to help relieve pain and stiffness. This method was developed in the USA as recently as the 1970s by Joseph Heller who, as well as using the physical applications to resolve poor posture, places much emphasis on the psychological aspects and emotions associated with stress.

- **Tragerwork** is another therapy developed in America. It involves a system of rhythmic rocking movements, allowing the body to gently stretch and release tension. Milton Trager, himself a sufferer of chronic back pain, devised the technique aimed at using transcendental meditation to achieve a state of relaxation to improve mobility.

- The **Bowen** technique, devised in Australia in the 1950s, uses soft rolling massages of certain muscle groups with the intention of stimulating the electrical impulses in the nervous system to release tension in the muscles.

Key points

- There are many different complementary therapies available that are used to treat back pain.

- Evidence to support the effectiveness of these therapies is patchy, and contentious for some.

- Choosing the right one – if any – for you should entail:

  - First seeking advice/getting a diagnosis from your family doctor.

  - Researching the pros and cons of the therapy that sounds right for you thoroughly.

  - Seeking recommendations and case histories from friends and family.

- Before deciding on the practitioner you want to treat you, check:

    - What training, qualifications and experience does he/she have?

    - Is he/she a member of a professional body?

    - Is he/she covered by professional indemnity insurance?

    - What will the total cost of treatment/instruction be, taking into account anticipated numbers of sessions?

- Be clear at the outset what you should expect (what changes and how quickly).

- Remember at all times that if the treatment causes pain and/or makes your back problem worse you should STOP.

References

Ernst E. Adverse effects of spinal manipulation: a systematic review. *JR Society of Medicine* 2007; 100 (7): 330-338.

Ernst E. Is reflexology an effective intervention? A systematic review of randomised controlled trials. *Medical Journal of Australia* 2009; 191(5): 263–266.

Ernst E. Vascular Accidents after neck manipulation: cause or coincidence? *International Journal of Clinical Practice* 2010; 64 (6): 673-674.

Furlan AD, van Tulder MW, Cherkin D, et al. Acupuncture and dry-needling for low back pain. *Cochraine Library* 2010; DOI:10.002/14651858.CD001351. pub2.

Graves S, et al. Influence of Pilates-based mat exercise on chronic lower back pain. *Medicine & Science in Sports & Exercise* 2005; 37 (Supplement 5):S27.

Jha A. Chiropractors may be no use in treating back pain. *Guardian* 9th November 2007.

Licciardone JC. Responding to the challenge of clinically relevant osteopathic research: efficacy and beyond. *International Journal of Osteopathic Medicine* 2007; 10 (1): 3-7.

Linde K, Allais G, Brinkhaus B, Manheimer E, Vickers A, White AR. Acupuncture for migraine prophylaxis. *Cochrane Library* 2009; DOI: 10.1002/14651858.CD001218.pub2

Little P. Randomised controlled trial of Alexander technique lessons, exercise & massage for chronic & recurrent back pain. *British Medical Journal* 2008; 337: a884.

Loeser J, Melzack R. Pain: an overview. *The Lancet* 1999; 353: 1607-1609.

Madsen MV. Acupuncture treatment for pain. *British Medical Journal* 2009; 338: a.3115.

National Institute for Health & Clinical Excellence. Early Management of Persistent Non-specific Low Back Pain. Guideline 88: London, 2009.

Rubinstein SM. Adverse events following chiropractic care for subjects with neck or low back pain: do the benefits outweigh the risks?' *International Journal of Clinical Practice* 2008; 64(6): 673-7.

Williams NH. Cost utility analysis of osteopathy in primary care. *Family Practice* 2004; 21 (6): 643-650.

Chapter 15

Motivation

Motivation to exercise cannot be taught or read in a book. In many cases, just like a New Year resolution, the intention exists but quickly wanes if the anticipated benefits are not soon realised. Sometimes the lifestyle change which is necessary can become inconvenient or time-consuming.

Not everybody finds it easy to accept a change of behaviour, especially one that requires a conscious application to every action and task in an already busy lifestyle. From standing in a queue, to washing the car or just relaxing with a drink at the end of the day, the deliberate effort to correct poor posture can easily be lost amongst the plethora of other important thoughts and actions. Even in industry, where there is formal training, knowledge of the legal requirements and even the provision of specific equipment to safeguard the welfare of employees, it is acknowledged that complete implementation of safer strategies may still be ignored in favour of speed and old hazardous techniques. 'I've done this for years and I don't have a back problem,' is the most commonly heard excuse.

Back pain and back injury, as already explored, do not generally just affect the sufferer. The moral argument that our own incapacity is also likely to affect the lives of others does not usually inspire us to work at our general fitness. That is, until the painful consequences of our actions are evident. The financial implications of a possible prolonged period of absence from employment is also hardly likely to be foremost in our minds when we are in the garden pulling at the start cord of the lawn mower. But the bottom line in many cases is that back pain is avoidable.

Obviously, self-interest is the strongest incentive to initiate change. Pain can be both a good motivator as well as a deterrent. For some, the need to take positive action in order to gain relief is motive enough, but for others the very thought that movement may increase discomfort ensures it is best left alone – at least for the time being.

The fact is, the spine was made to move and the more it moves, the healthier it will be. We know that Olympic athletes do not develop their strength and agility overnight. It takes years of dedicated exercise and training to enable them to achieve their superb levels of fitness. Fortunately, such extreme effort is not required in order to develop a level of fitness that gives us the flexibility and muscle strength to carry out our daily activities in a way that will prevent the occurrence or return of back ache. The only training required is to have sufficient self-discipline to always apply the correct lifting techniques that will avoid the risk of injury.

It may seem like a paradox, but the more exercise you take, the more energy you have for everyday life. It can give you a real buzz, make you feel good, and greatly improve your stamina. This, added to your refined and toned body, can even become addictive. Many exercise programmes and therapies that concentrate on stretching muscles and ligaments work on the benefits for soft tissues and the release of stress and tension.

Necessary as this aspect of physical health is, it is also vital to remember that the health of our bones should not be ignored. The bones of our skeleton are not just a hard, solid frame onto which the rest of our body clings. Bone is a living and changing part of our bodies and requires just the same attention to its strength and density, particularly as we age. The strength of our bones is proportionate to the demands made upon them. Therefore, if the skeleton is subjected to frequent high-impact work, such as squash or running, the bones are stimulated to increase in strength in order to manage the demand. Conversely, a purely sedentary lifestyle will allow the bones to lose some of their solidity, so that they become weaker and more prone to fracture.

Regular exercise has been proved to both prevent and control many of the common conditions associated with aging. Osteoporosis (porous bones which become fragile and weak) can to some extent be prevented by high-impact or weight-bearing exercise such as running, energetic walking or dancing. Even one or two short sessions of this type of exercise a week can greatly improve bone density.

For those recovering from back pain and who normally enjoy regular energetic exercise, the question most often asked is, 'When can I start again?'

Motivation for such people is already keen and they need little encouragement. For the rest of us, however, when life gets back to normal our busy lifestyle once again overwhelms any good intentions we may have had when the pain was in existence.

A positive approach to our general health does not really have to take more than a few minutes out of a day or impose rigid regimes that become difficult to maintain. If necessary, make small changes to your diet, such as reducing the amount of coffee, and foods high in sugar and salt. An awareness of the need to consume sufficient essential vitamins, such as A, C and D, will help enormously to maintain strong and healthy bones, muscles, ligaments and nerves which are vital for the health of your back.

Once the back pain has gone, try to keep as fit as possible. Take moderate daily exercise, graduated at first according to your age and limitations, and extend over time. As your level of fitness improves, this will not only strengthen your physical wellbeing but will give you more stamina that will resist any feelings of lethargy which may have dogged you in the past. This does not have to be formal exercise that takes up a lot of time – just getting off the bus one stop early and walking that distance will help.

Even after the last twinges of back pain have completely disappeared, take a few minutes to repeat those stretching and strengthening exercises contained in this book, especially those which you felt gave you the most help when the pain was bad. By persistently strengthening the muscles which control the area that gave you the initial problem, this will help to protect you from any future accidents or unavoidable strains to that part of your back.

The exercises described in this book have been formulated to offer a basic and constructive programme to give both relief and positive improvement for non-specific back pain. There are, of course, very many other techniques available and I hope my brief description of the methods of both orthodox and complementary therapies have helped you decide whether one of these treatments is for you.

You might like to consider contacting an association or organisation which specialises in exercises relevant to back pain (see Appendix). Half an hour spent with like-minded people who have suffered similar problems in their own lives will not only help you to maintain your motivation but will be an opportunity to make new friends. Both Pilates and Yoga offer courses not just for back pain but for complete health.

I know that it can be very demoralising when back pain, with no apparent cause, is deemed not to exist. The pain is very real and debilitating but in many cases can be overcome and may even present an opportunity to consider your lifestyle and attitude to everyday tasks. I hope that the tips and suggestions contained in this book have been helpful and will go some way to relieving and avoiding those very unpleasant symptoms. I wish you well.

Key points

- Not everybody finds it easy to make changes in their lives.

- Self-motivation can be difficult but small changes can make a big difference.

- Just remember back pain can affect you and your loved ones both socially and financially.

- If nothing else, make a deliberate effort to improve your posture...

- And ensure your diet includes calcium and vitamins A, C and D for strong bones and muscles.

- The spine was made to move and the more we exercise it the healthier it will be.

- The strength of our bones is proportionate to the demands made on them.

- Weight-bearing exercise can control the onset of osteoporis.

- Even small amounts of exercise can help – don't be overambitious.

- Try to maintain the exercises described in this book.

- Consider contacting a back pain association or organisation appropriate to your need.

Appendix

Resources and references

Professional Bodies and Associations

UK

Association of Reflexologists
27 Old Gloucester Street
LONDON WC1N 3XX
Tel: +44 (0)1823 351010
www.aor.org.uk

BackCare (National Back Pain Association)
16 Elmtree Road
Teddington
Middx. TW11 8ST
Tel: 020 8977 5474
www.backcare.org.uk

British Acupuncture Council
63 Jeddo Road
London W12 9HQ
Tel: 020 8735 0400
www.acupuncture.org.uk

British Chiropractic Association
Blagrave House
17 Blagrave Street
Reading
Berkshire RG1 1QB
Tel: 0118 950 5950
www.chiropractic-uk.co.uk

Chartered Society of Physiotherapy
14 Bedford Row
London WC1R 4ED
Tel: +44 (0)20 7306 6666
www.csp.org.uk

General Osteopathic Council
176 Tower Bridge Road
London SE1 3LU
Tel: 020 7357 6655
www.osteopathy.org.uk

International Federation of Reflexologists
78 Edridge Road
Croydon
Surrey CRO 1EF
Tel: 0870 879 3562
www.intfedreflexologists.org

Institute for Complementary Medicine
PO Box 194
London SE16 7QZ
Tel: 020 7237 5165
Email: info@icmedicine.co.uk
www.i-c-m.org.uk

The Pilates Room
69a Waldemar Avenue
Fulham
London SW6 5LR
Tel: +44 (0)20 8780 1308
www.thepilatesroom.org.uk

Research Council for Complementary Medicine
27a Devonshire Street
London W1G 6PN
Tel: 020 7935 7499
Email: info@rccm.org.uk
www.rccm.org.uk

Society of Teachers of the Alexander Technique
1st Floor, Linton House
39-51 Highgate Road

London NW5 1RS
Tel: 0845 230 7828
Email: enquiries@stat.org.uk
www.stat.org.uk

Tenscare Ltd
81 East Street
Epsom
Surrey KT17 1DT
Tel : 01372 3434
www.tenscare.co.uk

Yoga for Health Foundation
Ickwell Bury
Northill
Biggleswade
Bedfordshire SG18 9EF
Tel: 01767 627271
Email: admin@yogaforhealthfounda-tion.co.uk
www.yogaforhealthfoundation.co.uk

USA

American Back Society
2648 International Boulevard Ste #502
Oakland CA 94601
USA
Tel: +1 510 536 9929
www.americanbacksoc.org

American Chiropractic Association
1701 Clarendon Boulevard
Arlington
Virginia 22209

Tel: +1 (0)703 276 8800

www.acatoday.org

American Naturopathic Association

1413 King Street, First Floor

Washington DC 20005

Tel: +1 (0)202 682 7352

www.anma.org

American Physical Therapy Association

1111 North Fairfax Street

Alexandria, VA 22314-1488

Tel: +1 703 684 2782

www.apta.org

Australia

Australian Healthcare & Hospitals Association

PO Box 78

Deakin West, ACT 2600

Australia

Tel: 02 6162 0779

www.ahha.asn.au

Australian Osteopathic Association

11 Chatswood

NSW 2057

Australia

Tel: +61 2 9410

www.osteopathic.com.au

The Australian Physiotherapy Association

Level 1, 1175 Toorak Road

Camberwell VIC 3124

Australia

Tel: +61 3 9092 0888

www.physiotherapy.asn.au

Reflexology Association of Australia

PO Box 366

Cammeray

NSW 2062

Tel: 1300 733 711

www.reflexology.org.au

New Zealand

National Reflexology Association

PO Box 38860

Wellington 5045 MSC

New Zealand

www.reflexology.org.nz

New Zealand Society of Physiotherapy

PO Box 27 386

Wellington 6141

New Zealand

Tel: +64 4 801 6500

Webmaster@physiotherapy.org.nz

The Osteopathic Society of New Zealand

PO Box 647

Rangiora 7440

New Zealand

Tel: +64 3 313 5086

www.osnz.org

Other helpful websites

General Council for Massage Therapy
www.gcmt.org.uk

Association of Traditional Chinese Medicine
www.atcm.co.uk

American Association of Oriental Medicine
www.aaom.org

Australian Acupuncture & Chinese Medicine Association Ltd
www.acupuncture.org.au

American Massage Therapy Association
www.amtamassage.org

The Massage Association of Australia
www.maa.org.au

The Association of Massage Therapists & Holistic Practitioners
www.ampwp.org

Massage New Zealand
www.tmanz.org.nz

General Chiropractic Council
www.gcc-uk.org

Further reading

Daley D. *Body Moves* Cico Books, London, 2010

Kavanagh W. (2004) *Massage Basics* London: Hamlyn, 2004. (Extracted from *Home Health Massage* New York: Octopus, 2002.)

Parker S. *The Body Book* London:Dorling Kindersley, 2007.

Schwichtenberg M. (2007) *Yoga For Beginners* Oxford: Meyer & Meyer Sport (UK) Ltd, 2007. (Translated from *Yoga für Einsteiger* Aachen, Germany: Meyer & Meyer, 2006.)

Selby A. *Banish back pain the pilates way*. London, UK: Thorsons, 2003.

Sherwood P. *Your Back, Your Health* London, UK: Random House, 2007.

Trainer G, Alexander T. *Back Chat*. London, UK: Aurum Press, 2011.

Worby C. *Everything You Need to Know About Yoga*. Newton Abbot, UK: David & Charles, 2004.

Young J. *Complementary Medicine*. Chichester, UK: John Wiley, 2007.

Index